TEA CLEANSE DIET

Boost Your Metabolism by Introducing Tea Into Your Lifestyle

(How to Use Herbal Teas to Cleanse Your Body)

Scott Craver

Published by Sharon Lohan

© **Scott Craver**

All Rights Reserved

*Tea Cleanse Diet: Boost Your Metabolism by Introducing Tea Into Your
Lifestyle (How to Use Herbal Teas to Cleanse Your Body)*

ISBN 978-1-990334-40-5

Legal & Disclaimer

The information contained in this book is not designed to replace or take the place of any form of medicine or professional medical advice. The information in this book has been provided for educational and entertainment purposes only.

Table of contents

Part 1

Introduction

Every day millions of people, all over the world, consume tea on a daily basis. For some, it is an elixir that aids in digestion and for others; it is a tonic that keeps them awake. No matter what the reason, tea is the most widely consumed beverage in the world.

Invented in China, tea was regarded as a drink of the gods. It was then introduced to the Portuguese in the 16th century, who then took it to Britain in the 17th century.

Ever since, each country has its own signature tea like the Chai tea in India, which uses a blend of spices, and the Chinese tea, that uses thickened sweet milk.

Tea, as a warm beverage, helps in keeping people awake no doubt but also helps in cleansing the body in many ways. It clears away all the toxins from inside the body and promotes good health.

In this book, we will read on how teas can help in cleansing your body. We will look at the different types of teas, and also the recipes that you can use to avail good health.

Let us begin.

Chapter 1: What Is Tea Cleanse And Other Faqs

First and foremost, I wish to thank you for downloading this book and hope you have a good time reading it. In this first chapter, we will look at the different questions that get asked on the topic and answer them to help you understand it better.

What is tea?

Tea is a hot beverage that is brewed using water and crushed tealeaves. Tealeaves are picked from tea plants. They are generally grown in hilly regions as the climate suits the crop well. Tealeaves are laden with anti-oxidants, which make them extremely useful for our bodies. Apart from anti-oxidants, it is also laden with many vitamins and supplements that help in boosting our body's illness fighting capacity. Tea is prepared all over the world and each country has a different recipe.

Are they used straight from plants?

No. They are generally processed in factories where they are dried and powdered. The raw leaves cannot be used as they will not release a flavor and need to be oxidized. Even if you dry it yourself, you might not be able to avail its full benefits. Factories generally send the leaves through several processes before packaging it to be used by the end consumer. In some cases people do use the leaves as is. It will depend on the quality of the leaves. If you get your hands on the freshest leaves then you can probably brew a mild yet enticing brew. You might not be able to prepare tea made with milk and only the one where the leaves release a mild flavor.

What is a tea cleanse?

Tea is used as a tonic to cleanse your body. You can brew tea and consume it on a regular basis to cleanse your body from the inside. Through the course of this book, we will look at how tea can help in cleansing your body and the different preparations that you can brew in your kitchen. We will look at all the internal organs that get cleansed with these herbal and Ayurvedic teas.

Who is it for?

Tea cleanse can be adopted by anyone and everyone. Those interested in cleansing their bodies from the inside out can take it up. There is no age limit and right from young children to elders, everybody can take up tea cleanse to cleanse their body. Tea cleanse is generally prescribed for those people who wish to eliminate toxins from their bodies and put their health back on the right track.

Is regular tea good enough?

No. You have to consume certain special teas in order to lose weight. These teas are mostly prepared using special tealeaves that are designed to help in cutting down on the toxins in the body as also reducing the fat cells. You have to consume these teas on a regular basis unlike regular tea that you skip every now and then. Through the course of this book, we will look at the different teas that you can consume to help with weight loss and elimination of toxins from your body.

What is it used for?

Tea cleanse is mainly used to cleanse the internal organs of the body. It is used to eliminate the toxins that can build inside the body over the years. It is also used to aid in weight loss and improve metabolism. You can use tea cleanse to improve your immunity and longevity as well. We will read in detail the different ways in which tea can help you in chapter 2 of this book.

Is it really effective?

Yes. A tea cleanse is extremely effective. There is scientific backing to prove that the internal organs greatly benefit from tea cleanses. There are also many testimonials available on the Internet where people who have used the tea cleanse describe their experience and also illustrate how it helped in improving their health. Although there is no scale to measure the improvement, your overall health can greatly improve when you take up the tea cleanse.

How long before results show?

That depends on your body type and how serious you are about the cleansing. If you are really determined to lose weight then it will easily happen for you without having to put in too many efforts towards it. But if you are taking it lightly or casually then it might take some time for the results to show. You have to remain enthusiastic and take the routine up seriously. Many people start experiencing positive results within a day or two while others take a week or a month. You will have to feel it from the inside and that will only happen if you are seriously following the tea cleansing routine.

Will they vary?

Yes. The results generally vary, as it will all depend on the person's body type. If you are trying to lose a lot of weight, then it will take some time. If you wish to lose only a little weight, then it might come about soon. Usually, losing weight is quite easy during the first few weeks and then it starts getting tough owing to the body getting adjusted to the diet. However, by persisting with it and remaining determined to lose the weight. You will be able to see positive results.

Is there any evidence/ scientific backing?

Yes there is. Various research studies have been conducted on the effects of teas on the body. Almost all point to how teas can be used to cleanse the body from the inside out and also reduce weight. These studies have been conducted on a variety of people to know how tea actually affects each body type. The results have all been scientifically approved and you are sure to experience positive benefits by making use of tea.

What will I need for it?

You will require tea leaves for it. There are many types to choose from like green tea, black tea, Kombucha etc. I'm sure you have heard of these teas and might have also savored some of them in your life. Each one will help your body in a different way. We will look at all of them in detail in chapter 6 of this book. You can either choose all of them or try them individually and stick with the one that suits your body the best.

Where can I find it?

You can find them in powder form or in tealeaf form in any departmental or grocery store. You can also find them in specialty stores like traditional Indian stores or Chinese medicine stores. It is also easily available on the Internet where you can order it in bulk. But if you are buying combination teas then ensure that is a good brand. You must also check the list of ingredients in the tea to see if all of it is organic and healthy.

How long should I continue the tea cleanse?

In general, most cleanses last a week. You are required to brew the teas and consume them on a regular basis. But if you want to continue with for longer, then you can do so. It is important for you to treat it as a body cleansing system and continue with it for a long time. If you can replace your regular tea with it then it will be for the best. But it can also be used as a supplementary drink that you can drink along with your regular, daily beverage.

Will it be expensive?

No. Although some of these teas are exotic, they might not necessarily be expensive. You have to look for a good brand to buy and use them on a regular basis. These teas are generally bought in bulk, which will reduce the overall costs. You can order them online and avail their full benefits. If you are worried about the prices then it is best to prepare a budget and then follow it to avoid overspending. You will have the satisfaction of picking tea that is good for your health and also remaining within budget.

Should I try all?

Ideally, yes. It is best that you give all the different teas a try and then find the best one that suits you. Some people have different teas to serve a different purpose. Don't worry, they will not all combine into one and will work separately on your body. You have to try to have them during different times of the day like having green tea in the morning, hibiscus tea in the evening, yerba tea in the night etc. With time, you will be able to know the right combination.

Can I quit anytime?

Yes. If you are continuing with the tea for a long time and wish to quit then the choice is fully yours. There is no compulsion and if you feel that your body is now thoroughly cleansed then you can stop consuming the tea. There are no apparent side effects but if you are bored of the tea then you can either switch to another one or stop with it completely.

Are there any precautions that I should observe?

Yes. There are a few precautions that you will have to observe when you wish to consume any of the herbal or Ayurvedic preparations. As you know, everybody has a different body type and it is hard to generalize. How your body might react to a certain ingredient might be different from how another person's body will react to it. So, it is important to do a little trial and error to see if the diet is working well. If you already are aware of any allergies then you should steer clear of the ingredients that are not suitable for your body. We will look at them in in the last chapter of this book where everything is explained in detail for your convenience.

These are some of the common questions that get asked on the topic of Tea Cleanse and hope you found the answer to yours.

Chapter 2: What Tea Cleanse Helps With

Tea cleanse is a great way to cleanse your body from the inside out. In fact, it is said to be much more effective than consuming fruits on a regular basis. In this chapter, we will look at the various ways in which it cleans your body.

Weight loss

Tea cleanse in weight loss. In fact, it is this reason why most people opt for a tea cleanse. Obesity is now a growing trend and the only way to beat it is by modifying our diet. In fact, not taking quick action can cause you to develop unnecessary illnesses brought about by obesity. The herbal teas will aid in cutting down fat and help you attain a slim and trim body. It also assists in digestion, which further enhances the body's capacity to lose weight and remain slim. We will look at this aspect in detail in chapter 3 of this book.

Cleansing

Tea as you know helps in cleaning your body. You will feel much healthy and fit by consuming the different teas on a regular basis. These cleansing teas are aimed at restoring a balance inside the body. As you know, there are both acids and neutrals in your body. It is important for you to maintain this balance and one way of doing so is by consuming healthy teas from time to time. We will look at the different digestive tea recipes in this book that will help you remain fit and healthy.

Appetizer

Tea works both ways. Not only does it help in a person losing weight but also assists in increasing appetite. So for all those looking to increase their weight or wishing to increase their appetite, tea can do wonders to you. It will assist in also cleansing your stomach and increasing your hunger.

Food cravings

If you are trying to get over any food cravings like junk or processed food cravings, then tea can help in reducing it. Of course you cannot expect a miracle. It is not like you will drink tea today and your food cravings are gone tomorrow. It will take some time and your body will have to adjust to it. If you suddenly stop doing something that your body is used to then the habit will return in no time at all, and with twice the force. So, you have to take it a little slow and see to it that your body is adjusting well to the new habit.

Digestion

Tea contains tannic acid that helps in breaking down the food particles. This can then be easily digested by the body. Many people use tea as a digestive and drink it after having a meal. You too can do the same and help your body digest the different foods that you eat. Once you get accustomed to it, your body will start demanding the tea and will be able to remain fit and healthy for a long time.

Longevity

It has been scientifically proven that tea helps in increasing a person's life span. That is, it aids in a person availing good health and living a fuller life. Teas are full of anti-oxidants that help in fighting free radicles and increases cell health. You must be aware of Chinese men and women living long lives and living well past 100 years. Most of them attribute their long life to drinking tea. They consume the tea on a daily basis and try to drink 2 to 3 times a day.

Common illnesses

Given how we lead stressful lives and undertake unnecessary tensions, we end up falling sick quite often. Add to it the ill effects of pollution and potent germs doing the rounds, it is quite difficult for us to ward off illnesses such as common coughs and colds. But, with the regular consumption of tea, it is possible to ward all off these and lead a healthy life. It is not possible to completely eliminate the germs of course and the most that you can do is reduce the number of times that you fall sick in a month.

Grave Illnesses

Apart from regular coughs and colds, it is also possible to limit or mitigate some illnesses that are chronic in nature. They might have been brought about by obesity or some other such cause. The more important part is for you to ward them off and the best way to do is by consuming tea on a regular basis. This tea is not your regular milky tea and an herby concoction, which we will look at in detail in a future chapter of this book.

Immunity

Regular consumption of tea helps in increasing immunity. You will have the strength to fight off illnesses and also maintain a strong digestive system. You will have reduced episodes of bad stomach and despite consuming food prepared at restaurants you will be able to maintain a calm stomach. It is known to contain chemicals that are helpful in increasing your body's capacity to resist disease causing bacteria and keep unwanted ailments such as common colds and coughs at bay.

Hair

Teas help in adding shine to your mane. It will work from the inside out and increase your hair's tensile strength. I'm sure you would have read green tea as an ingredient in some of the shampoos that you use. That is because green tea is like an elixir for hair. It improves the texture as well. You can in fact douse a couple of green tea bags in warm water and allow it to diffuse for a while and then use it as a tonic to wash your hair. You will see that your hair has turned soft and shiny.

Skin

Teas also help in keeping your skin healthy and glowing. Drinking tea regularly will help in increasing the elasticity in your skin. That will prevent it from becoming loose and developing wrinkles. It also imparts a unique glow to the skin. If you suffer from dark circles below your eyes then you must place a couple of green tea bags in water and then place them over your eyes. Allow them to remain there for a few minutes and then wash with cold water. Do this for around 2 weeks and you will see that the dark circles are slowly disappearing and the skin around your eyes is tightening up a bit. You can also add in a little green tea into your face pack if you wish to avail its benefits and tighten your whole face.

Energy

Tea helps in keeping your energy levels up. The caffeine in it is what helps in increasing your energy and keeps you fit. You will not feel lazy and have enough energy to last a busy day. You will also have the capacity to take on the chores at home and not feel tired easily. If you have the morning blues then they can easily be chased away by consuming tea.

Sleep

If you suffer from insomnia or face trouble sleeping then tea can help solve the problem. By consuming chamomile tea on a regular basis, you can effectively fight away the problem and fall asleep easily. Apart from chamomile, there are also other concoctions that you can brew and consume to fall asleep better. We will look at these teas in a bit.

Hormones

Teas help in regulating hormones. During puberty, most people's hormones get affected and they start functioning irregularly, the best way to solve this problem is by consuming teas on a regular basis. These need to be herbal teas that make use of ingredients that are good for the overall body.

These are just some of the good effects of tea on your body and are not limited to just these. There are a lot more of them, which you will only realize once you start consuming tea on a regular basis.

Chapter 3: Tea Cleanse And Weight Loss, Detoxification And Digestion

How does it help with weight loss?

Tea is a bush that mostly grows in Asian regions. Its scientific name is Camellia Sinensis and is used to prepare a hot brew. Tea has many uses but one of the most sought after use is its ability to help in weight loss. Tea has the capacity to cut down on the fat cells in your body. It contains caffeine and EGCG, which help in improving metabolism. This elevated metabolism helps in digesting food faster and eliminates the build-up of fat. Amongst all the teas, green tea is the most preferred one to assist in weight loss.

What are the toxins?

There can be many toxins in our bodies. Some of the most common ones include methane, carbon monoxide, metals like zinc, mercury and chemicals such as ammonia, chlorine etc. These toxins can be quite poisonous and need to be eliminated from our bodies. They can tamper with our organs and cause our bodies to function at a slower pace. They can also confuse our bodies and cause it to think adversely. These can exist in babies as well and is not only something that adults have. In fact, babies will have it more as their bodies will be young and unable to combat these toxin-causing germs easily.

Where they exist?

These toxins generally exist inside our bodies. They mostly attack organs such as kidney, liver, gut and intestines. They will start tampering with these organs and cause them to dysfunction. There will always be a line of defense but given the type of stressful lives that we lead, it will not always be possible for our bodies to fight these away easily. They can also seep into our blood stream and end up affecting most of the organs inside our bodies. They also affect our colon to a large extent.

How do they come about?

There are 4 main categories through which these toxins come about and they are as follows.

Air: Air can contain a lot of chemicals that come about through pollution. Right from methane to carbon monoxide, vehicles can emit all types of toxins, which get absorbed into our bodies. Apart from vehicle emissions, they also come in through factory emissions. If you are a smoker, then the number of chemicals in your body will be much higher and will mostly settle in your lungs.

Water: Water is laden with chemicals and that is no secret. Right from ammonia to chlorine to bleach, there are many chemicals that are toxic for our bodies. There are also some antigens that can be present which can cause bad stomachs, liver and gut issues etc.

Some factories end up dumping toxic chemicals into rivers that supply water to our homes as well.

Food: Most of the junk and processed foods that we consume are laden with dangerous chemicals. They will add in preservatives and also artificial colors and substances that can cause our bodies to weaken. These toxins are also capable of altering our hormones and might cause them to misbehave.

Environment: The environment can also end up releasing lots of toxins that can get absorbed by our bodies. There are chemicals that get released from the cleansing products that we use. Mercury is also predominantly present in the air that we breathe and that is also quite toxic for our bodies.

Why they should be cleansed?

These chemicals should be eliminated from our bodies in order to maintain basic health. Although most of them are eliminated through sweat, urine and feces, some will always be left behind. It is important to help the body in eliminating these toxins. The best way to do is by consuming cleansing drinks from time to time. These teas will have the capacity to clean out the toxins from the organs. If you wish to regain your strength and lead a healthy and fit life then it is best to cleanse your body off of these toxins on a regular basis.

How to cleanse them out?

As was mentioned earlier, the best way to clean them out is by consuming herbal and Ayurvedic teas. The ingredients present in these teas will help in eliminating the toxins from the body. The teas will also aid in improving immunity, which will help the body natural fight, the toxins off. We will look at some of the best detoxifying tea recipes later in this book.

Cleansing kidney

The kidney is one of the main organs in our body. It is like a sponge that absorbs all the toxins and eliminates them through our rectus. So, it is important for us to keep our kidneys clean. Herbs such as celery root and hydrangea can help a great deal in keeping the kidneys healthy and functioning optimally for a long time. Dandelion and parsley can also be used for the same purpose but it is important to distil the tea properly before consumption.

Cleansing gut

The gut is an organ that assists the liver and cleansing our bodies. If there is a complex compound that the liver is unable to process then it will promptly send it to the gut. However, thanks to the consumption of processed and junk foods, our gut can stop functioning optimally and a condition called gut rupture can come about. It is important to prevent it and strengthen our gut. The best way to do is by consuming a tea made from watermelon seeds and marigold flowers. These can be steeped in green tea, strained and consumed. Regular consumption will ensure that your body is fit enough to combat any of the chemicals.

Cleansing liver

The liver is an organ that helps in breaking down the compounds in food. It is given the role of getting rid of toxins from food and distributing the important nutrition to the rest of the body. The liver also has a line of defense known as Kupffer cells, which help in absorbing free radicles and also fighting away antigens. The best herb to cleanse the liver is mint as it helps in strengthening the cells. You can prepare a tea using the leaves and consume on a regular basis.

Cleansing stomach

Our stomach can become a storehouse for toxins and it is important for us to cleanse it from time to time. Consuming black tea on a regular basis helps in relieving flatulence and keeping your stomach lining intact.

Cleansing colon

Our colon is what takes all the toxins from our bodies out. Lemon juice is an effective ingredient that you can use to cleanse your colon. The juice can be added into any of your teas and consumed regularly. Green tea is also extremely effective in cleansing your colon and will aid in keeping the cells free from cancer.

Chapter 4: Types Of Teas And Herbs Used

When it comes to tea, there are many varieties that are available. In this chapter, we will look at the different varieties of teas and also some of the natural ingredients that are used to in combination with these teas.

Regular Tea

Regular tealeaves are better known as Camellia Sinensis. Predominantly grown in the eastern region of India, this tea is said to be extremely rich in anti-oxidants. A majority of Indians brew a tea made using these leaves that are boiled in water along with spices and mixed with milk. This tea is said to help ward off regular ailments like cough and cold and will also help boost immunity. You can easily buy this type of tea at a store or also find it online. You must look for the variety that offers a combination of small and long leaves. The same tea is interpreted in different ways in other Asian countries. The Chinese make use of thickened condensed milk for their tea and people in Middle East make use of a tea ball that is immersed in boiling water to flavor the tea.

Black Tea

Black tea is a traditional Chinese preparation and uses the tealeaves Camellia Sinensis. It comes from the same bush as regular tea. It goes through a different process, which lends it the black charred tinge and also imparts a different taste. There are many varieties of black tea including Assam tea, Darjeeling tea, Nepal tea etc. These are prepared by steeping the tealeaves in hot water for a long time or until they release a deep black color. Nothing else is added to the tea and is consumed as is. Those that have acquired its taste can only enjoy this type of tea.

Green Tea

Green tea is one of the most widely consumed tea in the world and gained popularity in the last decade as awareness of its goodness spread. Green tea is full of an anti-oxidant known as catechins. These catechins work wonders on a person's stomach and also aid in increasing immunity. Green tea is also extremely effective in helping the body lose weight. It cuts down on the fat cells in the body and makes for a great diet supplement. In fact many people consume green tea along with every meal as it helps in breaking down the foods that are consumed.

Kombucha

Kombucha better known as Kombu is a type of fermented black tea that is known to benefit people's livers. Liver is responsible for producing an important bodily fluid known as bile and so, it is important to keep it healthy. You can do so by consuming Kombucha tea on a regular basis. People also add a little to their food in order to predigest it and then consume the food, as it will be easily digested. However, you must exercise precaution when using it and use it only in the recommended dosage.

Flowering Tea

Flowering tea refers to the leaves and the flowers that are tied together and used to prepare tea. This type of tea is quite mild and imparts a floral flavor. It is important to not boil such teas too much and allow them to remain in water for only a few minutes before serving. It is a traditional Chinese technique of consuming tea and is generally had in the mornings. There are many variations of this tea and although most people consume it sweet, some people add in a little salt to their flowering tea to balance out the flavors.

Peppermint

Peppermint is an herb that is used for many purposes. Right from cold to coughs, conjuring up a brew using green tea and peppermint leaves helps in healing from these ailments faster. Peppermint is also used to avail relief from stomach problems such as gas, bloating and general discomfort. It helps provide instant relief from irritable bowel syndrome. Those women who experience pain during periods can also make use of this herb in order to avail instant relief. It also helps in calming down acidity and improves over all digestion.

Chamomile

Chamomile is the other ingredient that is most commonly used in brewing teas. It is a flower that is rich in a chemical, which induces sleep. Many people use it as a sleepy time ingredient and brew a concoction that is used to serve as a sleeping aid. It has chemicals that help in inhibiting stress and also help in curbing anxiety. Chamomile helps in reducing flatulence and provides instant relief from flatulence. If you are having a mild headache or migraine then try sipping on some chamomile tea for relief.

Dandelion

Dandelion leaf and flower are used to brew teas. They help in improving digestion and are also used to treat a mild case of diarrhea. So if you are having a mild case of it, then it is best to make use of dandelion tea and avail instant relief. That makes it a great ingredient to carry outdoors as well to quickly remedy an upset stomach. Dandelion has a mild fragrance and a milder taste. It has the texture of a fibrous flower and is dried and pound.

Hibiscus

Hibiscus is the other best flower that I used in making tea. Hibiscus is a red or white flower, which is perennial in nature. They contain chemicals that help in eliminating toxins from the body. You will be able to lead a healthier and fitter life by consuming hibiscus tea on a regular basis. Hibiscus is mostly just plucked from the plant and added to the tea mix. The entire flower is safe to consume including the petals, stamen, and the calyx. There are many other colors of hibiscus available and you can pick the one that is available to you. It is also a good idea to make use of its leaves. Wash them thoroughly and tear them roughly to be added to the tea. This is a great way to improve hormonal balance.

Holy Basil

Holy basil is a great herb to use and prepare tea. Holy basil is a perennial plant that is mostly grown in Asian countries. It is one of the healthiest herbs in the world. It contains chemicals that help in combating regular coughs and colds. Holy basil has an amazing mild taste that helps in keeping the breath fresh. So tearing a few leaves and adding to your morning tea will help you maintain fresh breath all through the day. Holy basil also produces seeds that are great for your body. You can incorporate these seeds in your diet.

Ginger

Ginger is one of the most commonly used ingredients in Asia and is generously added to Chai. Ginger is a root vegetable that is rich in many vitamins and is said to be an extremely healthy ingredient to consume. It is used as medicine as well. It helps in digestion and promotes the growth of healthy bacteria in the stomach. It also assists in releasing unnecessary toxins from the skins and helps add a glowing tinge to it. Ginger has a very sharp taste that can seem a bit strong for first time consumers. But its sharp taste is what makes it an effective medicinal ingredient and can intensify the flavor of the tea. Ginger provides instant relief from sore throat and coughs.

Mint

Mint leaves cool the body down and is much preferred for their sweet taste. They can be added to pretty much any kind of tea and will enhance the flavor. Mint contains chemicals that help in cooling the body down. By consuming mint leaves on a regular basis you will be able to increase your body's capacity to fight off disease causing germs and also increase your immunity. It is as easy as adding a leaf or two to your tea and stirring it around. You can eat the mint leaves too!

Lemon

Lemon is used to flavor tea. Right from green tea to black tea, lemon is used to enhance the flavor and also add in nutritional benefits. As per Harvard school of public health, a little lemon added to tea helps in increasing immunity and also strengthens your teeth and bones. It fights away free radicles and ensures that your body remains strong for long. It is also a powerful ingredient that helps in controlling the level of sugar in your body and can aid in curbing the onset of diabetes.

Spices

Many spices are used in making tea, especially chai tea. Right from cloves to cardamom to pepper, all the spices are ground and added to tea. These are great to not only flavor tea but also instantly releases heat. This heat helps in warming up the body and awakens it from the inside. The spices are said to contain chemicals that improve immunity. In fact, many yogis advice consumption of spiced tea as it also aids in relieving a bad stomach and might provide relief from flatulence and indigestion. One of the most widely used spices is cinnamon. Cinnamon is a great spice as it helps in increasing the body's digestive capacity. It can be powdered and added to teas and then strained. Don't worry if you eat some of the cinnamon bits, it is full of flavor and will leave a woody taste behind. Another spice is the star anise. This too is full of flavor and will assist in cutting down on the amount of fat cells in your body. Without fat cells, you will be able to cut down on your chances of getting fat.

Lemon Balm

Lemon balm is an herb that is quite popular amongst the elders. It has the tendency to reduce wrinkles and promotes skin elasticity. So regular consumption of lemon balm tea will help you look younger for longer. It also supports the liver thereby reducing the occurrence of skin issues. It also strengthens hair roots and makes it soft and silky. Lemon balm has a strong flavor, which can help in releasing sinus and also aids in reducing cough and sore throat.

Fennel

Fennel seeds are extremely nutritious and cool the body down. Fennel seeds are also rich in vitamin C, which helps in strengthening your immunity. It also helps in keeping bad breath at bay and increases the production and release of good bacteria in your stomach. It is also a diuretic; so, it will help in eliminating the build-up of fluids in your body. Fennel is also a great herb to use to fight obesity and maintain a slim and trim figure. Many women also drink fennel tea to correct their hormones and fight ailments such as PCOS.

Cumin

Cumin is a spice that is extensively used in Asian cooking. It is known as a cure all in many traditional texts and is an elixir for stomach ailments. It helps in curbing diarrhea and also assists in improving digestion. A little cumin tea every morning will ensure that coughs and colds are kept at bay. Cumin is great to avail relief from stomach pain, especially if caused by bacteria. Cumin tea also helps in preventing bad breath and will leave behind a fresh taste in your mouth.

Caraway Seeds

Caraway seeds are great for digestion. Just a few seeds are enough to cleanse your stomach and liver. It also provides relief from flatulence and cramps caused by periods. It is generally used in combination with coriander seeds.

Carom seeds

Carom seeds are another healthy seeds to incorporate in your teas. Carom seeds are slightly spicy yet full of flavor. They will help you cut down on bad breath and also digest foods. If you have had a heavy meal then you can consume a tea made from carom seeds, as it will help in breaking the food down.

Turmeric

Turmeric is a root that is ground into a fine powder and added to tea. It has anti-bacterial and anti-viral properties that make it ideal for your body. It will help in increasing your immunity and also assist in digestion. But it is important to use it in limited quantity as it can upset your stomach if taken in excess.

These form the different ingredients that are generally used in preparing medicinal teas.

Chapter 5: Myths About Tea

When it comes to teas, there are many myths that surround it. People know that tea is a health drink cum an energy booster but carry around many myths in their minds about it. In this chapter, we will burst the different myths and help you understand the topic a bit better.

Tea Is Bad For Health

This is one of the most prominent tea myths in the world. People assume that tea is bad for the body as it can cause many internal effects like acidity. But as we already saw in previous chapters, tea is one of the healthiest drinks in the world. You can avail many health benefits and remain healthy and fit for a long time when you consume tea on a regular basis. Yes, it can cause acidity but only if you get the combination of ingredients wrong. We will look at how you can brew tea the correct way in the next chapter.

Tea Will Kill Sleep

There is a myth that says tea will kill your sleep and not allow you to avail a good night's sleep. This is only a myth and there is no truth to it. The main ingredient that causes you to stay awake is caffeine. Although tea generally has more caffeine than coffee, you will not have to stay up at night if you drink a cup in the morning. Caffeine works in different ways with different people and it will be hard to generalize. If you think you are staying awake at night due to tea then it is best to not consume it after 2 pm.

Tea Is Expensive

There is a myth that tealeaves are expensive and you will not be able to afford it for long. But that is not true. Tea costs just as much as coffee and in fact, even lesser. So don't worry about the price, as you will not have to spend a lot of money on buying your tealeaves. You can set yourself a budget and go as per it. You will see that you can buy many varieties of teas within a small budget. Buying them in bulk online will further help you save on the overall costs.

Tea Is Boring

This myth has been doing the rounds for some time now. People assume that coffee is the only drink that can be made interesting but the same extends to tea as well. We will look at many interesting recipes further in this book, which will tell you how interesting tea really is. You will see that the tea you brew is quite tasty and sure to make you change your mind about it. You can experiment as much as you like with tea and come up with newer and newer recipes.

Tea Is Useless When Boiled

Many people believe that tea will lose its power when boiled in hot water. The water will strip it off of its nutrients and cause it to be mild. But this is only a myth. If the water removes the nutrients then they will be dissolved in it and you will use the same to brew your tea. So, you will be consuming the nutrients and they will help you maintain a strong and fit body. There is also no rule that you should use boiling water alone to brew your tea.

Re-Boiling Tea Will Make It Taste Bad

Another myth states that re-boiling tea will make it taste awful. Again, this is only a myth. Tea will not taste bad if you re-boil it. It might taste a little different but not bad. But if it is possible for you to discard the tea and prepare a fresh batch then that is also a good option. The taste of fresh tea is unbeatable and you will be addicted within no time.

Organic Tea Is The Best

This is another myth that needs to be busted. It is understood that organic tea is good for health but you have to be careful when buying it. You cannot buy whatever you get in the market and must do your research on the brand. There might be some frauds out there that will combine chemicals and call it tea. So, you should try and read on the brand and buy the best. You can check out the brands and their testimonials on the Internet. The same extends to Ayurvedic and herbal teas. All of them will help you improve your health no doubt but you have to be 100% sure before consuming it.

Green Tea Is The Healthiest

Yes, green tea is quite healthy no doubt but is not the healthiest of the teas. You can choose from other teas as well like black tea and regular tea. All of them will provide you with health benefits and they are not limited to green tea alone. If you wish to avail full benefits of the teas then you will have to pick the freshest leaves and use them to brew the tea.

Black Tea Is Stronger Than Green

Many believe that black tea is stronger than green owing to its rich black color. But this is not true. Just because green tea is pale green does not mean it is not strong. Both are equally strong and you will see that the teas are providing you with equal health benefits. You have to brew both the right way and we will look at that in detail in a future chapter of this book.

Adding Spices Will Make The Tea Weird

No. This is a misconception. It is understood that spices and tea may sound like a weird idea but the two go hand in hand and they will enhance the flavor of tea. The spices will give it a dense and woody flavor. This type of tea is most common in Asian countries. The spices will also help in relieving cold and cough symptoms. So, adding in a blend of spices to your tea is a great idea if you wish to increase its flavor and health benefits.

Sugar In Tea Is Harmless

Many assume that just a teaspoon or two of sugar in their daily tea is harmless. That is a big myth. The sugar in your tea is enough to increase the level of sugar in your blood. So, don't think the little sugar will not get noticed by your body. It is best to either choose a sweetener or pick honey.

These form the different myths that surround teas and hope you had yours answered efficiently.

Chapter 6: Right Way To Brew Tea

As you know, there are many ways in which tea is brewed. But did you know that there are certain right and wrong ways for teas to be brewed? In this chapter, we will look at the different ways in which you can brew tea.

Black Tea

Black tea is one of the easiest teas to prepare and yet the most powerful. You can avail, many health benefits from black tea and here is how you can prepare it.

1-cup water

1 rounded teaspoon black tea leaves

Start by boiling the water. You can use an electric kettle or place the water in a saucepan. The water should bubble up. Now add around 1 tablespoon of this water inside the cup that you wish to brew the tea in and warm he cup up. Once it is warm, you should throw the water out. Now add in the 1-teaspoon of black tea leaves to the hot water and cover it. You can now allow it to steep for 3 to 5 minutes or more, depending on how strong you want it to be. Once the time is up, you can strain it into the cup and serve it. You can also make use of an infuser to serve the same purpose. This tea is best had as is or you can also add in some milk or squeeze in lemon to enhance its flavor. You can also add in some sweetener to it if you wish.

Green Tea

Green tea is also just as easy to prepare as black tea. Here is how you can prepare it with ease.

1-cup water

1-teaspoon green tea leaves

Start by adding the water to a saucepan and allow it to come to a boil. Once it reaches around 180 degrees, you can add one teaspoon to the glass and discard it once the cup is hot. Now, add in 1 teaspoon of the leaves to the water and allow it to steep for 3 to 5 minutes. Steeping it any longer might cause the tea to develop a bitter taste. Once done, you can strain and add it to the cup. You can also prepare the tea in an infuser if you like and follow the same procedure. It is best to not add anything to green tea and consume it as is. Some people add sugar to it but that will take away some of its health benefits. In some Chinese traditions, people first brew black tea and pour it into the cup and then discard it before adding in the green tea to it. This is said to help enhance the health benefits of green tea.

Regular Tea

Regular tea is made using tealeaves and milk. It is one of the most preferred teas in the world and what many people drink in the mornings to have a boost. Let us look at how you can prepare it.

5 tablespoons water

2 teaspoons regular tealeaves

3/4ths cup milk, skimmed or full cream

Sugar to taste, or honey

Start by adding the water to a saucepan and allow it to come to a boil. Now add in the tealeaves and simmer it for 2 minutes. Once the tea leaves release their flavor, you can add in the milk and allow it to come to a boil. Add the sugar or honey to the glass and then strain the milk mixture into it. Give it a stir and serve hot. This tea tastes best only when milk is added to it.

Thai Tea

Thai tea is another tea that is great to taste and simple to make. Here is a quick recipe.

1-cup water

1-tablespoon milk

1-tablespoon condensed milk

2 tablespoons Thai tea laves

Sugar, optional

Start by placing the water in a pot or saucepan and brining to a boil. Once it boils, you can add in the milk and tealeaves and allow it to come to a boil. Simmer it for a few seconds. Add the condensed milk to a cup and then strain in the tea mixture. Give everything a good mix and serve hot. This tea tastes best when the sweet condensed milk is added to it. Since the condensed milk is sweet, it is best to avoid adding in any extra sugar to it. If you wish to make iced tea then you can skip adding in the milk and condensed milk and add in crushed ice.

The Chinese too make a similar tea but they will only use the condensed milk and not the water and milk. So their version will be extremely sweet and quite thick.

These form the different ways in which you can brew tea. We already looked at the different equipment that you will need for tea and you can buy and use them.

Chapter 7: What Makes Tea Good?

Tea is a great tasting drink and millions of people savor it all over the world. But what if there is a way to enhance the flavor of tea? What if you could increase its color and flavor? Will that not be a great thing? Well surely it would! In this chapter, we will look at the different aspects to consider with tea in order to enhance its flavor and richness.

Leaf Size

The very first thing to consider is the size of the leaves. The tea shrub grows flat conical green leaves that are picked and processed. The plant will produce both long ones and short ones, which will be present on the same plant. The shorter leaves will provide you with an enhanced flavor and are therefore much preferred to the longer ones. The shorter are also widely bought by big tea companies, as they will impart a great flavor. As you know, when the tea is picked and dried, they will shrivel up. Once they do, you will still be able to tell whether it is a short leaf of a long leaf. Although it is a good idea to make tea using the short leaves, you have to use a blend of both long and short to avail the best flavor. You will see that the tea you brew is much more colorful and strong in flavor and capable of improving the overall taste of tea.

Leaf Dust

Many countries make use of leaf dust to brew tea. This dust refers to the tiny bits of tealeaves that are left behind after the best leaves have been packed. This dust is said to produce a very strong flavor, as the concentration of caffeine will be quit high in them. You too can make use of it as it will help you produce strong tea and more importantly, will prove to be cost effective. You can look at the size of the leaves as it is generally mentioned on the pack.

Leaf Color

The leaf color will also have an impact on the tea's flavor. Those teas that are pale in color will come from leaves that are pale themselves. These will not carry a strong flavor and will impart the tea a faint flavor. The next are dark colored leaves, which will impart the tea a strong flavor. You have to pick dark leaves that are almost black in color if you wish to make strong tea.

Leaf Type

The type of leaf used to prepare the tea is also important. The tealeaves that are plucked are all tender shoots of the plant. As was mentioned before, most good quality tealeaves are picked in the 2 leaves and 1 bud pattern. This is said to contain the most flavor. This unit as a whole is processed to produce the tea powder. You can use it to prepare the best tasting tea. Apart from this, you can also choose the one that is made from short leaves. This was discussed in the previous segment.

Season

The season when the leaves are plucked also makes a difference. March to November is seen as the best time to pluck these leaves. It is said that the plants reach their best during these months and you have to pluck them in batches. The first flush in plucked between March and April. The second flush between May and June, the third flush between July and August and the autumn flush between September and November.

Country

As you know, the weather differs from country to country. There are some countries whose weather is great for tea. The tea that is grown in Asian countries is said to be the best in the world. The weather in these countries favors the growth of the tea plant. You must have heard about Darjeeling tea. That refers to tea that comes from a place in the Northeastern region of India known as Darjeeling. The weather in Darjeeling is said to be extremely beneficial for the growth of tealeaves. These plants are mostly grown on hills. There are many estates there and each one plucks the leaves on a regular basis. Apart from Darjeeling, Sri Lanka is also famous for growing tea.

The Water

Next, the quality of the water also determines the quality of the tea. So, you have to pick between spring water and tap water. It is not a good idea to make use of distilled water. That water will cause your tea to taste flat and might also cause it to develop a metallic taste. So, you should choose quality water to prepare the tea.

Steeping Temperature

The steeping temperature also plays a part in enhancing the flavor of the tea. It is best to maintain the temperature between 180 degrees and 220 degrees centigrade. You can either buy a thermometer to check the temperature or buy an electric kettle that will tell you the temperature of the water. Both will help you prepare the best tea.

Steeping Method

The method that you use to steep the leaves will also have an impact on the taste of the tea. Some prefer to dip the tea bags while some place them in the kettle. Some add the leaves to the boiling water while others add the water to the leaves. Each one will produce a different taste. You will have to perform a little trial and error to find the best technique that can be employed to prepare the tea. In general, it is a good idea to steep the tea bags in the kettle to avail an enhanced flavor.

Bags

Many people don't realize that it is not such a good idea to make use of tea bags. The tealeaves in it would have oxidized and the flavor they will impart will not be that good. Still, if you wish to use these bags then it is best to make some by yourself instead of buying them from stores.

These form the different things to consider while making the best tea. They will all come together to give you the best flavor.

Chapter 8: Tea Making Process

As you know, tealeaves go through many processes before they can be consumed. In this chapter, we will look at the different processes that these leaves are sent through.

Plucking

The very first thing is to pluck the leaves from the plant. These leaves are to be plucked carefully and only experts are allowed to do it. The plucking expert knows how to pinch the bottom of the leaves and pulls it upwards without damaging it. They are provided with baskets on their backs where they throw the plucked leaves. They will know which leaves are tender and which ones have matured. Some experts will pluck both mature and tender leaves in order to give the tea a certain characteristic. If you have the chance to visit a tea estate then you can volunteer to pluck some of the leaves and understand how it is done.

Quality

The next step is where the leaves are all sent through quality checks. Here, the experts will look at the leaves and pick the best ones and discard the bad ones. Quality check is extremely important, as only the best quality leaves will help in producing the best tea. Those leaves that have holes or have insects will be discarded at this level. The numbers are quite staggering as out of a 100 kilograms of tealeaves that are generally plucked, around 20 to 25 kilograms are sent to the next process. So, almost 80% of the plucked tealeaves are rejected.

Weight

The next step is to have all the leaves weighed. In a day, a regular tea picker will be able to pluck several basketfuls of tealeaves. So, it is important to weight each one. They are batched as per their size and then weighed. Only the ones that will be used are weighed. The ones that are discarded are usually sent to other factories or exported. Many countries import rejected tealeaves and prepare the powders. It works out cheaper by the kilogram.

Transport

The weighed leaves are then packaged and transported to the factories. They are generally batched into groups and the fresh ones and the mature ones are all shipped separately. Generally, these leaves take a long time to reach the factories, as most tea estates are not placed around factories.

Drying

The next step us known as drying or withering. This is one of the most important processes as it is important to make the leaves liable. The leaves are all laid out on large sheets and dried under the sun. Some big factories have special dehydrating machines that blow hot air and dehydrate the leaves. It takes around 24 hours for these leaves to dehydrate completely. This process also makes the leaves soft and will easily be processed in the next step.

Rolling

The next step is known as rolling. Rolling refers to breaking down the different cells in the leaves. This helps in the leaves releasing a unique flavor, which is the most important part of the tea making process. This step also helps in initiating the next level of processing, which is known as the oxidizing. This process takes around a day to finish. Since tea factories are always functioning, one batch or the other will always be in the rolling machine.

Oxidizing

Oxidizing is possibly the most important process of preparing tealeaves. Oxidizing refers to exposing the leaves to the oxygen in the air. This helps in releasing the different flavors in the tea. The tea leaves change color from green to black, which is an indication of the oxidation. The tea that is oxidized the most will appear the darkest and is better known as black tea. Depending on the variety that the factory is aiming at, the tealeaves will be oxidized. Some prefer to oxidize it until it turns light brown and some will wait for it to go completely black. The latter will take much longer than the former owing to which, most factories prefer the former option.

Firing

The next process is known as the firing process. This is where the tealeaves are prepared for the final process. This involves drying them completely. This drying is important as it seals in the flavor of the tea. Also, it helps in preserving the leaves for a long time. They will not go bad, as there will be no moisture left. The companies use heavy-duty blowers to blow and eliminate the moisture from the leaves.

Sorting

Next, the different leaves are all sorted out. As you know, there are long leaves, short leaves and the dust. These are all sorted and separated into different batches. They are placed into different machines in order to aid in the next process. This sorting process is generally manually done or might be mechanized. It depends on the scale of the factory.

Tasting

The next process is known as tasting. Experts taste the tea and grade it. The best tasting teas are given the highest ranking and the ones with the mild flavor are given the lowest. This step is also taken to ensure that the tea is uniform and hat the whole batch is good to go. Apart from tasting the tea, they will also look at the quality of the leaves and decide whether the batch stays or needs to be discarded.

Packing

Finally, these leaves are all packed into different boxes. Once they are packed, they are shipped to the different markets.

These form the different steps that are taken in processing the tealeaves.

Chapter 9: Herbal Teas

Herbal teas are one of the most sought after in the world of healthcare. Made from fresh herbs, these teas are full of nutrients. In this chapter, we will look at some of the best herbal teas that you can try at home and avail good health.

Raspberry Leaf Tea

Calories 2

Ingredients:

- 1 teaspoon dried raspberry leaves
- 1 cup water
- 1 green tea bag

Method:

- Add the water to a pan and allow it to boil.
- Add the raspberry leaves to a cup.
- Add in the green tea bag to the same cup.
- Pour the hot water into the cup and cover it.
- Allow it to stand for 5 minutes without disturbing it.
- Uncover it and pour it through a strainer.
- Drink the tea hot.
- Don't add in any sweetener.
- This tea is great for women suffering from hormonal imbalances. It is prescribed to those that suffer from endometriosis, PCOS and other hormone related issues.

Elderberry Tea

Calories 2

Ingredients:

- 2 cups water
- 1 green tea bag
- 2 tablespoons dried elder berry leaves
- ½ teaspoon turmeric powder
- 1 teaspoon honey

Method:

- Start by adding the water to a pan and bringing it to a boil.
- Add in the elder berries and lower the heat.
- Add the tea bags to a heat resistant pitcher.
- Add in the berry water and allow it to steep for 5 to 10 minutes.
- Strain the tea and if it has gone a little cold then you can boil it once again.
- Add in a pinch of turmeric and a little honey and serve hot.
- This tea is great for those suffering from flu. And it will also help in strengthening the body after a viral fever.

Tea For Sore Throat

Calories 2

Ingredients:

- 2 cups water
- 1 green tea bag
- ½ cup sage leaves
- 1 teaspoon crushed cloves
- 1 cinnamon stick, ½ inch

Method:

- Start by adding the water to a saucepan and bringing it to a boil.
- Add the sage leaves and tea bag to a heat resistant pitcher.
- Add the cloves to the water and simmer for a minute.
- Add the water to the pitcher.
- Allow it to stay for 5 minutes.
- Strain it into a glass and you can add in the cinnamon stick to stir it around.
- This tea will provide instant relief from a sore throat brought on by cold. If the sore throat is really bad then it is advisable to drink this tea twice a day.

Holy Basil Tea

Calories 2

Ingredients:

- 1 cup fresh holy basil leaves
- 2 cups water
- 1 green tea bag
- 1 tablespoon honey

Method:

- Start by adding the water to a saucepan and bring it to a boil.
- Add the green tea bags to a heat resistant pitcher.
- Add the water and allow it to steep for 5 minutes.
- Add in the holy basil leaves and leave it for 10 minutes.
- Strain this mixture and heat it again.
- Add in the honey and serve hot.
- This tea will help in improving your immunity. You can serve this tea to children as well and if they are really young then you can skip the part with the green tea bag.

Nettle Tea

Calories 3

Ingredients:

- 1 cup nettle leaves
- 2 green tea bags
- 4 cups water
- 1 tablespoon honey

Method:

- Add the water to a pan and bring to a boil.
- Add in the nettle leaves and simmer it for 15 minutes.
- Strain it and add the water to another pan and bring to a boil.
- Add it to a glass along with honey and serve hot.

- This tea is great for detoxification of your systems.

Black Tea With Rose

Calories 2

Ingredients:

- 2 cups water
- 1 black tea bag
- 1 cup rose petals

Method:

- Add the water to a pan and bring it to a boil.
- Add the black tea bag to a pitcher.
- Add in the water and allow it to steep for 5 minutes.
- Add in the rose petals and let it stand for 10 minutes.
- Strain the tea and you can reheat it before serving.
- This tea is great for all those looking to detoxify their body and avail a rosy glow.

Chapter 10: Ayurvedic Teas

Ayurveda is a traditional Indian medicinal system that makes use of fresh spices and herbs. In this chapter, we will look at some of the Ayurvedic teas that you can prepare and consume on a regular basis.

Ginger And Turmeric Tea

Calories 2

Ingredients:

- 1 tablespoon ginger
- 1 teaspoon turmeric
- 1 cup water
- 1 Indian spice blend tea bag
- 1 teaspoon honey

Method:

- Start by adding the water to a saucepan and bring it to a boil.
- Add the eta bag to a heat resistant pitcher.
- Add the ginger and turmeric to the boiling water and then simmer it for 10 minutes.
- Once it boils, add it to the pitcher and allow it to steep for 10 minutes.
- Strain the mixture and boil it once again.
- You can add in a spoon of the honey and serve the tea hot.

- If you are unable to find the Indian spice tea bags then you can prepare your own. To prepare the tea bag mix together tea leaves along with a couple of cloves, 1 black cardamom pod, 1 teaspoon black pepper corns, ½ inch cinnamon stick and a few green cardamom pods.
- This tea is great to avail relief from coughs and colds and will do wonders to those looking to lose their weight.

Chili Tea

Calories 2

Ingredients:

- 2 cups water
- 2 green tea bags
- ½ red chili
- 2 tablespoons honey

Method:

- Start by boiling the water in a saucepan.
- Add the tea bags to a pitcher.
- Add the chilly to the water.
- Add in the honey and mix well.
- Pour the tea into a glass and serve hot.
- This tea will help in cleansing your digestive tract.

Cumin And Caraway Tea

Calories 1

Ingredients:

- 2 cups water
- 2 black tea bags
- 1 tablespoon cumin seeds
- 1 tablespoon caraway seeds
- 1 tablespoon coriander seeds

Method:

- Start by adding the water to a saucepan and bring to a boil.
- Add the cumin seeds, caraway seeds and coriander seeds to a small pan and dry roast it for 5 minutes.
- Add it to a coffee bean grinder and create a fine powder.
- Add the mix to the boiling water and allow it to simmer for 10 minutes.
- Add the tea bags to a pitcher and pour the water.
- Allow it to stand for 5 minutes.
- Pour it into a glass and serve hot.
- This tea is great for those women looking to avail relief from period cramps.

Spicy Chai Tea

Calories 2

Ingredients:

- 1 cup almond milk
- 1 Indian chai tea bag
- 2 tablespoons honey

Method:

- Start by boiling the almond milk in a saucepan.
- Add the honey to it and mix well.
- Add the tea bag to a cup.
- Add the sweetened milk and serve hot.
- If you can't find the chai tea then mix teas leaves with cardamom, cloves and cinnamon, and steep it in boiling water for 5 minutes and then add in the sweetened almond milk.
- This tea is quite tasty and can be consumed on a regular basis.

Ashwagandha Tea

Calories 2

Ingredients:

- 1 tablespoon dried Ashwagandha (buy online)
- 2 cups water
- 1 black tea bag
- 1 tablespoon honey

Method:

- Add the water to a saucepan and bring to a boil.
- Add in the Ashwagandha and give it a mix.
- Boil it for 5 minutes and switch off the heat.
- Add the tea bag to the saucepan and allow it to steep for 5 minutes.
- Strain the mix into a cup and add in honey.
- Stir it and serve hot.

- This is a great tea for those looking to boost their sex drive. It is also good for those looking to increase their immunity.

Shankpushpi Tea

Calories 1

Ingredients:

- 2 tablespoons Shankpushpi leaves and flowers
- 2 cups water
- 1 tablespoon rose petals
- 2 tablespoons honey or sugar
- 1 pod cardamom

Method:

- Start by adding the water to a saucepan.
- Add in the Shankpushpi leaves and flowers.
- Allow it to boil for 5 minutes and then simmer it.
- Add in the rose petals and boil it further.
- Add in the cardamom pod and switch off the heat.
- Strain this mix and add to a glass.
- Add in the honey or sugar and serve hot.
- This drink is generally made for children as the herb helps in increasing memory power. If you wish to serve it to adults then you can add in a green tea bag.

Most of these ingredients can be easily found in departmental stores. But if you don't find them there then you can look for them online.

Chapter 11: Healthy Cold Teas

It is obvious that not everyone likes warm teas. So for all those interested in availing detoxification benefits through cold teas, here are some recipes.

Peachy Ice Tea

Calories 30

Ingredients:

- 2 Cups water
- 2 green tea bags
- 2 ripe peaches
- 2 tablespoons fresh mint leaves
- 1 teaspoon honey

Method:

- Start by adding the water to a pan and bringing it to a boil.
- To a heat resistant pitcher, add in the tea bags.
- Pour the boiling water into it and allow it to stand for 5 minutes.
- Remove the tea bags out and add in the honey into it.
- Give it a good mix until most of the honey dissolves.
- Allow it to cool to room temperature.
- Add in the mint leaves and bash them a little to help release the flavor.
- Add in pieces of the peach and stir.

- Place it in the freezer for 3 to 5 hours or add in crushed ice.

Lavender Tea

Calories 2

Ingredients:

- 2 cups water
- 3 green tea bags
- 2 teaspoons lavender blossoms (freshly picked)
- 1 large fresh lavender sprig, for decoration

Method:

- Start by adding the water to a pan and bring it to a boil.
- Place the green tea bags in a heat resistant pitcher.
- Add the boiling water to the pitcher and allow it to steep for 5 minutes.
- Remove the tea bags and allow the tea to come to room temperature.
- Now add in the lavender blossoms and crush using a muddler.
- You can add in some honey at this point if you like or leave it as is.
- Place it in the fridge for 3 to 5 minutes and then serve with a lavender sprig placed in the jar.
- You can also add in some ice cubes if you like.

Orange Surprise

Calories 4

Ingredients:

- 2 green tea bags
- 2 cups water
- 1 cup fresh orange pieces
- 1 teaspoon fresh orange peel
- 1 teaspoon lemon juice
- 1 tablespoon honey

Method:

- Start by pouring the water into a pan and bringing it to a boil.
- Add the green tea bags to a heat resistant pitcher.
- Pour in the boiling water and allow the bags to steep for 10 minutes.
- Remove the bags and allow the tea to reach room temperature.
- Add in the pieces of orange along with the lemon juice and honey and stir.
- Once it mixes, add in the orange peel and mix.
- Place in the fridge for 3 to 5 hours.
- Serve cold and add in crushed ice if needed.

Strawberry And Mint Tea

Calories 5

Ingredients:

- 2 green tea bags
- 2 cups water
- 1 cup fresh strawberries
- 1 teaspoon honey

- 2 tablespoons mint leaves

Method:

- Start by adding the water to a pan and bringing it to a boil.
- Add the tea bags to a heat resistant pitcher.
- Add in the water and allow it to stand for 5 minutes.
- Remove the bags and allow the tea to reach room temperature.
- Add in the pieces of strawberry along with the honey and give it a good mix.
- Turn it into the fridge or freezer for 2 to 5 hours.
- Add in the mint leaves before serving and can also add some mint leaves if required.

Coconut tea

Calories 10

Ingredients:

- 2 cups boiling water
- 1 green tea bag
- 1 cup coconut water
- ½ cup coconut flesh (fresh)
- ½ teaspoon mint leaves

Method:

- Start by placing the water in a pan and bring to a boil.
- Place the tea bags in a heat resistant pitcher.
- Add in the water and allow it to steep for 5 minutes.

- Remove the tea bag and let the tea cool down.
- Add in the coconut water along with the coconut flesh and stir until well combined.
- Turn it into the fridge for 3 to 5 hours.
- Serve cold with mint mixed in and a few ice cubes if needed.

Berry Tea

Calories 5

Ingredients:

- 2 tablespoons blackberries
- 2 tablespoons raspberries
- 2 tablespoons blackberries
- 2 green tea bags
- 2 cups water
- 1 teaspoon honey
- 1 teaspoon mint leaves

Method:

- Start by adding the water to a pan and bring to a boil.
- Add the tea bags to a heat resistant pitcher.
- Add in the boiling water and allow it to steep for 5 to 10 minutes.
- Remove the bag and add in the berries.
- The tea doesn't need to cool down.
- Use a muddler to crush the berries.
- Turn the drink into the fridge for 5 hours.

- Serve with mint leaves added in and also crushed ice.

Milky Ice Tea

Calories 15

Ingredients:

- 2 green tea bags
- 2 cups water
- ½ cup almond milk
- 1 tablespoon honey
- 2 tablespoons tapioca pearls (optional)

Method:

- Stat by adding the water to a pan and bring to a boil.
- Add the tea bags to a heat resistant pitcher.
- Add in the boiling water and allow it to steep for 5 minutes.
- Remove the bags and add in the honey and allow to cool.
- Add the almond mil and stir until well combined.
- Turn it into the fridge for 5 hours.
- Meanwhile, you can soak the tapioca pearls in water for 30 minutes or until they swell up.
- Add the pearls to a glass and top it with the coconut milk mix.
- You can serve it with crushed ice added in.

Rose Tea

Calories 2

Ingredients:

- 2 green tea bags
- 2 cups water
- Rose petals (all colors)
- 2 tablespoons honey
- 1 teaspoon crushed cardamom
- 1 cup water

Method:

- Start by adding the water to a pan and bring to a boil.
- Add the green tea bags to a heat resistant pitcher.
- Add in the water and allow the bags to steep for 5 minutes.
- Remove and add in the rose petals.
- You can use a muddler to crush it and help release the flavor.
- Add in the honey and mix until well combined.
- In a separate pan add in the ½ cup water along with the cardamom seeds.
- Once it to boil, turn off the heat and strain the water.
- Add the water to the rose mix.
- Turn it into the fridge for 5 hours.
- Serve cold and add in some crushed ice if needed.

If you are unable to find fresh rose petals then you can buy some dried ones as well. But ensure that they are food grade petals.

Chapter 12: Weight Loss Teas

Bilberry Tea

Ingredients:

- 1 cup hot water
- 1 bilberry teabag or 1 teaspoon bilberry tea powder
- ½ teaspoon sugar, optional

Method:

- Start by bringing the water to a boil in a saucepan.
- Add the tea bag to a cup and pour the hot water over it.
- Allow it to stand for 5 minutes.
- Now add in the sugar and mix until well combined.
- Serve hot.
- If you are using leaves then add the leaves to the boiling water and allow it to come to a boil.
- Add in the sugar, strain and serve hot.
- This tea is also good for the eyes and helps in cutting down on the risk of diabetes.

Star Anise Tea

Ingredients:

- 1 teaspoon black tea leaves or 1 black tea bag
- 1 cup water
- 2 whole Star Anise
- 1 teaspoon sugar, optional

Method:

- Start by adding the water to a saucepan and bringing it to a boil.
- Add in the tealeaves or the tea bags and allow it to step.
- Now add in the star anise to it and give it a good mix.
- The star anise should release its full flavor in the tea.
- Now strain the mix and pour into a glass.
- You can dissolve some sugar into it if you like.
- You can also dissolve some honey in it and serve.
- This tea is great for weight loss as it contains microbial that aid in digestion. Having this tea after a meal is surely going to help you cut down on excess weight.

Oolong Tea

Ingredients:

- 1 tablespoon oolong tea leaves
- 1 cup water
- Sugar optional

Method:

- Start by adding the water to a saucepan and allow it to come to a boil.
- Now add in the tealeaves and let it boil for 5 minutes.
- Now add in the sugar and mix until well combined.

- Strain this and serve hot.
- Oolong tea is famous for the different health benefits that it provides. It aids in cutting down on the level of cholesterol in the body and also improves overall health. Drinking this tea twice a day will help you remain fit and healthy for a long time.

Kombu Tea

Ingredients:

- 1 pack Ready to use Kombucha
- 1 cup water
- 1 green tea bag

Method:

- Start by bringing the water to a boil.
- Add in the green tea bag and let it infuse.
- Now add in the Kombucha and let it sit for 5 minutes.
- Strain the mix and consume.
- Kombucha is a type of fermented green or black tea that contains a type of yeast that aids in digestion. Drinking this tea regularly will help you remain slim and healthy. You might have to read the instructions supplied with the Kombucha to use it the right way.

Pu-Erh Tea

Ingredients:

- 1 teaspoon pu-erh tea leaves
- 1 cup water
- Sugar optional

Method:

- Start by bringing the water to a boil.
- Once it bubbles, add in the tealeaves and allow it to infuse the flavor fully.
- Once done, add in the sugar and mix until well combined.
- Serve this tea in a cup.
- Don't worry if tiny bits of the leaves escape from the strainer into the cup. They are harmless and will in fact provide you with greater health benefits.
- Pu-erh tea is widely consumed in china and is said to aid in shrinking the fat cells present in the body. These cells are what are responsible for your weight gain and shrinking them means shrinking your tendency of gaining weight.

Hibiscus Tea

Ingredients:

- 1 cup water
- 2 green tea bags
- 1 cup hibiscus flowers, red or white ones
- Sugar, optional

Method:

- Start by placing the water in a saucepan and bring it to a boil.

- Now add in chopped hibiscus flowers to it and allow the flavor of the flowers to seep into the water.
- Add the green tea bags to it and allow them to infuse.
- Let it remain for 5 minutes before removing the tea bags and straining the tea to be served in a glass.
- Hibiscus flowers are great for the body as a whole. It helps in reducing the fat in the body. It also helps in cleansing the blood and imparts glow to the skin.

Yerba Mate

Ingredients:

- Yerba mate tea leaves
- 1 cup water
- Sugar, optional
- Yerba mate tea gourd

Method:

- Start by adding the leaves to the gourd. If you don't have one then you can add it to a saucepan.
- Heat water in a pan and add it to the leaves. Alternately, pour the water in the saucepan and bring it to a boil.
- Use the stick/ straw to crush the leaves or stir the tea around.
- Once it heats, you can strain it and serve with the sugar.
- Yerba mate is a traditional drink and said to be extremely healthy. It is best consumed in the yerba mate gourd. It contains chemicals that help in

breaking down the fat content in the body. You can drink this tea in the mornings or the evenings.

White Tea

Ingredients:

- 1 teaspoon white tea leaves
- 1 cup water
- Sugar, optional

Method:

- Start by placing the water in a saucepan and bringing it to a boil.
- Now add in the tealeaves and allow them to release flavor.
- Once done, strain the mix, add in the sugar and serve.
- White tea is a special tea that is meant to help in weight loss. You can look for a good brand and buy it.

These teas must be had at least twice a day in order for them to work on your weight loss. You might have to indulge in some trial and error to find the tea that works best for you.

Chapter 13: Recipes Made Using Tea

Savory Recipes

Chickpea In Tea Sauce

Ingredients:

- 1 cup chickpeas or 1 can
- 1 tablespoon oil
- 2 garlic cloves, crushed
- 1 large onion, chopped
- 1 large tomato, chopped
- 1 teaspoon cumin powder
- 1 teaspoon paprika
- Salt to taste
- 2 cups water
- 2 tea bags
- Coriander to sprinkle

Method:

- Start by soaking the chickpeas in water overnight or rinse if using straight from can.
- Now heat the water and add the chickpeas to it and cook it until it is soft.
- In a pan, add in the oil, onions and garlic and mix until browned.
- Meanwhile, add the tea bags to a small cup of hot water and allow it to infuse for 3 minutes.

- Add the cumin, paprika, salt and tomatoes to the onion mix and stir until well combined.
- Now add in the tea and mix well.
- Once the chickpeas have softened, add them to the tomato mix and allow it to blend for some time.
- Serve hot with a sprinkling of coriander leaves on top.

Sweet Tea Rice

Ingredients:

- 1 cup milk
- ½ cup water
- 2 tablespoons condensed milk
- 2 tea bags
- 1 cup long grain rise
- 1 cup hot water
- 1 cardamom pod
- Sugar, optional
- ½ cup assorted dry fruits, roasted

Method:

- Start by adding the milk and water to a saucepan and allow it to boil.
- Meanwhile, add the rice to the hot water and cover it for 10 to 15 minutes or until it cooks 3/4ths.
- Once the milk heat, add the teabags and allow it to infuse for 5 minutes. You can also add in tealeaves for a rich flavor and the strain the mix.

- Once done, add in the condensed milk and give it all a good mix.
- Use a mortar and pestle to crush to the cardamom a little.
- Add this to the tea and give it a good mix.
- Now add the tea to rice and give it a good mix.
- Serve by sprinkling the assorted nuts on top.
- You can also chill this by placing in the fridge for a few hours.

Tea Chicken

Ingredients:

- 2 tea bags
- ¼ cup sugar
- 2 tablespoons salt
- 1 medium onion, chopped
- 1 small lemon, juiced and zested
- 2 garlic cloves, crushed
- 1 tablespoons thyme
- 1 tablespoon oregano
- 1 tablespoon rosemary
- Salt to taste
- Pepper to taste
- 1 whole chicken

Method:

- Start by preheating the oven to 400 degrees Fahrenheit.
- Grease an oven tray and set aside.

- Now place the tea bags, sugar, salt garlic, thyme, oregano and rosemary in a deep bowl and add in hot water.
- Allow everything to mix in well and remove the tea bags after 5 minutes.
- Now place the whole chicken inside the mix and allow it to coat completely.
- You can place the bowl in the fridge overnight to help the chicken coat well.
- Next, place the chicken on the baking tray and pour the lemon juice and rind over it.
- Place the onion pieces over it and place the tray in the oven.
- Allow the chicken to crisp up and then serve hot.

Tea Seafood

Ingredients:

- 2 tea bags
- 2 cup mixed seafood, prawns, shrimp, fish, crabmeat etc.
- 1 large lemon, juice and zest
- 2 garlic cloves, crushed
- Salt to taste
- Pepper to taste
- Parsley to sprinkle

Method:

- Start by steeping the tea bags in hot water and allow it to infuse.
- Remove it after 5 minutes.

- Now add in the lemon juice, zest and garlic and mix it until well combined.
- Add in the salt and pepper and mix well.
- Heat a saucepan and add in the seafood.
- Allow it to sauté for a few minutes until the seafood cooks.
- Serve with a sprinkling of fresh parsley on top.

Tea Infused Salad

Ingredients:

- 1 tea bag
- 1 large onion
- 1 large tomato
- 1 cucumber
- 1 tablespoon lemon juice
- 1 teaspoon olive oil
- 1 tablespoon mixed dried herbs
- 1 cup mixed beans, cooked
- Salt to taste
- Pepper to taste
- 1 tablespoon sugar
- Parsley to sprinkle

Method:

- Start by adding the tea bags to ½ a cup of hot water and allow it to infuse.
- Meanwhile, chop the onions, tomato and cucumber into tiny pieces.

- Add it to a bowl along with the salt and pepper and give it all a good mix.
- Now add in the mixed beans olive oil and dried herbs and mix.
- Pour the tea on top like a dressing and mix until well combined.
- Add in 1 tablespoon of sugar to the salad and serve with a sprinkling of snipped parsley leaves on top.

Meatballs In Tea Sauce

Ingredients:

- 1 pound ground meat, your choice
- 1 garlic clove, crushed
- 1 teaspoon oil
- 1 large onion
- 1 large tomato
- 1 tablespoon mixed dried herbs
- Lemon juice
- 2 tea bags
- Salt to taste
- Pepper to taste
- Coriander leaves to sprinkle

Method:

- Start by adding the oil to a pan along with the garlic and onion and allow it to brown.
- Steep the tea bags in hot water.
- Add the chopped tomatoes to the onion mix.

- Add the meat, salt, pepper and herbs to a bowl along with the lemon juice and make small balls out of it.
- Add the tea water to the tomato mix and stir until well combined.
- You must season the sauce as well.
- Now place the meatballs inside the sauce and cover with a lid.
- Cook it for 40 minutes or until cooked.
- Serve with a sprinkling of coriander leaves on top.

These form the different simple tea infused savory recipes that you can prepare.

Sweet Recipes

Tea tiramisu

Ingredients:

- 2 tea bags
- 2 cups sugar
- 1 tablespoon vanilla extract
- 2 cups mascarpone cheese
- 2 cups whipping cream
- 2 packs ladies fingers
- 2 tablespoon cocoa powder

Method:

- Start by boiling water and adding in the tea bags to it.
- Allow it to release color and flavor.
- Remove and discard the tea bags.
- Now add in the sugar to it and mix until well combined.
- Remove it from heat and allow it to cool down.
- Now place the cheese, vanilla extract and beat until well combined.
- In another bowl, add the whipping cream and beat until stiff peaks form.
- Now place half the lady's fingers at the bottom of a bowl and our half the tea mixture over it and allow it to soften.
- Next, place half the cheese mixture over it followed by half the cream.
- Place another layer of the lady's fingers and pour the rest of the tea mixture over it.
- Follow it with the cheese mixture and then the cream.
- Use a sieve to sprinkle the cocoa powder on top and place it in the fridge for 12 hours or overnight.
- Serve cold.

Tea Pudding

Ingredients:

- 2 tea bags
- ½ cup water
- 5 tablespoons condensed milk

- 1 cup sago pearls, soaked
- ½ cup mixed dry fruits, roasted
- 1 cardamom pod, crushed

Method:

- Start by boiling water and adding the tea bags to it.
- You can crush the cardamom pod and add it to the water.
- In another saucepan, bring the water to a boil and add in the sago pearls and allow it to go soft.
- Strain the tea and add to a cup. Add in the condensed milk and mix until well combined.
- Pour this over the sago pearls and mix well.
- Turn this into the fridge for 5 to 6 hours.
- Serve with a sprinkling of the dry fruits on top.

Tea Infused Cake

Ingredients:

- 2 cups boiling water
- 3 lemon tea bags
- 1 cup butter, softened
- 2 cups sugar
- 1/2 cup brown sugar
- 5 eggs, lightly beaten
- 3 1/2 cups all-purpose flour
- 2 teaspoons baking powder
- 1/2 teaspoon salt
- 1/4 teaspoon baking soda

Method:

- Start by preheating the oven to 300 degrees Fahrenheit.
- Add the hot water to a cup and add in the tea bags.
- Allow it to steep for 5 minutes.
- In a bowl, add in the butter, sugars and eggs and beat until light and fluffy.
- You can also beat the eggs separately if you want a light and airy cake.
- To a sieve, add the flour, baking powder, salt and baking soda and sieve it directly into the butter mix.
- Now fold this mixture in with gentle hands.
- Add in the tea and fold again.
- You can add in some lemon juice and rind if you wish to enhance the flavor of the cake.
- Now pour this mix into a greased baking dish and bake for 35 to 40 minutes.
- A skewer inserted in the center should come out clean.
- Allow to cool and serve.

Sweet Tea Bread

Ingredients:

- 2 tea bags
- 5 tablespoons condensed milk
- 1 tablespoon butter
- 4 slices bread
- 2 tablespoons assorted nuts, roasted and chopped

Method:

- Start by boiling water and steeping the tea bags for 5 minutes.
- Slice the bread into squares.
- Now place the butter on a pan and place the bread on top.
- Allow it to brown on both sides.
- Once done, place it on a plate.
- Now remove the tea bag and add the condensed milk to it.
- Mix until well combined.
- Pour this over the bread slices and spread using the back of a spoon.
- Sprinkle the nuts on top and serve.
- It can also be placed in the fridge for 2 to 3 hours before serving.

Biscuits With Tea Cream

Ingredients:

- 1/2 cup butter
- 1/2 cup sugar
- 1/2 cup brown sugar
- 1 large egg
- 1/2 teaspoon vanilla extract
- 1/2 tsp salt
- 2 cups all-purpose flour
- 1 teaspoons baking soda
- 1 teaspoon baking powder
- 1 cup milk chocolate chips
- 2 tea bags

- 5 tablespoons butter
- 5 tablespoons sugar

Method:

- Start by preheating the oven to 320 degrees Fahrenheit.
- Add the butter, sugar and vanilla to a mixing bowl and mix until well combined.
- Now add in the egg, flour and salt and mix until well combined.
- Add in the chocolate chips and mix well.
- Pick up a teaspoon full of the mix and roll it into balls.
- Place it on a greased baking tray and flatten it using your fingers.
- Place it in the oven for 10 minutes or until you see the cookies cook and turn brown.
- Meanwhile, steep the tea bags in ½ cup hot water and allow them to release flavor and color.
- Place the butter and sugar in a mixer and beat.
- Add in the tea mix and combine.
- Once the biscuits are done, remove and cool.
- Place a tablespoon of the cream on a biscuit and sandwich another one over it.
- Do the same with the rest and serve.

Tea Poached Pears

Ingredients:

- 5 black tea bags

- 4 cups boiling water
- 2 large pears
- ¼ cup sugar
- Vanilla custard, optional

Method:

- Start by placing the tea bags in the boiling water and allow it to steep for 5 to 10 minutes.
- Remove the bags and add in the sugar and mix until well combined.
- Now add this mix to a saucepan and bring to a boil.
- Add in the pears to poach it.
- Now lower the heat and cover it.
- Once the pears cook or soften, turn off the heat and keep it covered.
- Now remove the pears on a plate and pour some of the syrup on top.
- You can place a ladle full of the vanilla custard on top and serve.

These form the different sweet dishes that you can make using tea.

Chapter 14: General Precautions And Equipment Needed

Most of the teas mentioned in this book are safe for consumption. However, there are some precautions that you must observe while using some of these ingredients and they are as follows.

Pregnant Women

It is important for pregnant women to exercise a little precaution while consuming any of these teas. It is best to consult the doctor first to know if the ingredients are safe to be consumed. It is best to prepare the teas at home using fresh ingredients instead of buying ready-made ones from stores. Dandelion, Chamomile and ginger are not safe during pregnancy and should be avoided. If you happen to consume it by mistake then it is important to consult your doctor at the earliest. However, holy basil is a great pregnancy herb to consume as it helps in building immunity.

Elders

It is important for the elders to speak with their doctors before consuming any tea. Some of the ingredients might not suit their bodies as it might take a long time to digest. Herbs such as nettle and dandelion might not be suitable for elders. However, elderberry is a great ingredient for elders and will keep them fit and healthy for a long time. Men suffering from prostate issues can consume saw palmetto tea.

Children

It is not advisable to give children tea of any kind as it contains caffeine. Caffeine is good for the body no doubt but can cause energy levels to spike. This is especially bad for children suffering from ADHD and must be avoided at any costs. However, it is a good idea to cut out the tea part from the recipes and give children herby warm concoctions. It will help in boosting their immunity and also improve their digestive capacity.

Medications

If you are consuming any medicines for diabetes then it is important to avoid the teas containing peppermint. You must also avoid ginger and try to consume more of the teas containing lemon or lemon balm. Both of these will help in brining the sugar level in your body down.

Allergies

If you are allergic to any of these herbs or spices then you must avoid consuming them. If you feel any discomfort after consuming the tea then you must cease consuming it and consult a doctor immediately. If you are taking any diuretics or blood thinners then avoid consuming dandelion tea and try to consume more of the fennel teas.

It is extremely important to exercise precaution when consuming nettle. It can sting and you should handy the leaves with care. If you do experience a stinging sensation then you should rub it with ice cubes to avail relief.

Remember that these mere precautionary advises and should not deter you from adding cleansing teas to your regular diet.

Equipment Needed To Prepare The Teas

Heat resistant pitcher

A heat resistant pitcher is generally made of glass and can easily be bought online. Just ensure that you are buying good quality pitcher from a trusted brand. Remember that no heat resistant pitcher can tolerate extreme temperatures and you must never add in any liquid that has gone beyond its boiling point. If the pitcher develops a crack then it means that it is not heat resistant and you must change it. Most of these pitchers are made of clear glass. Some of these can directly go on a flame as well and buying such a pitcher will make it extremely easy for you to prepare the teas.

Muddler

A muddler is generally made of wood or glass. You can use it to crush some of the ingredients that you add to your tea. A good quality muddler will be sturdy and made of grainy wood. If you are unable to find a muddler then you can also make use of a spatula to help you crush the ingredients.

Strainer

A strainer is what you use to strain your tea. A good quality strainer is generally made of metal like stainless steel. It is best to avoid plastic ones as the heat can melt it to a certain extent. You can buy a good strainer online.

Tea ball

A tea ball is traditional Middle Eastern equipment that is used to help prepare tea. The ball is made of metal and opens in the center. You can place the tealeaves there and close the ball. It comes with a chain that you use to lower the ball into hot water. Once your tea is prepared, you must remove the ball out. The ball is washable and can be used over and over again. You can also add in spices and herbs along with the tealeaves.

Infuser

An infuser is a device that you can use to prepare tea instantly. It has a valve in the center where you can add in the leaves and any other herb or spice and water goes around it. You then close the lid and wait for the ingredients to infuse. If it is an electric infuser them the water will boil inside it. If it is a non-electric one then you must add hot water to it. Once the tea is ready, you can pour it out into a glass.

Electric kettle

Buying an electric kettle will make it very easy for you to prepare the teas. You can add water to the kettle and boil it quickly.

Tea bag covers

Tea bag covers can be purchased in bulk online. They are used to fill in tealeaves and herbs. You can look up recipes online and create your own tea bags. You can also refer to the recipes mentioned in this book and prepare your tea bags. You must close it tightly and staple it to prevent any spill outs. You can also add a tag at the end to know what it contains.

Chapter 15: Tea For Body Cleansing

It is obvious that you can use tea for your external body as well. Here are some things that you can do to prepare natural cosmetics and toiletries with your tea.

Eye Bags

Puffy eyes are one complaint that most women have. Eyes get puffy due to many reasons such as lack of sleep or dehydration. Here is a simple eye bag that you can make and use to avail relief from your puffy eyes. You will need tea bag covers, 2 teaspoons green tea leaves and 1 teaspoon lavender flowers. Pack all of these in the tea bag and steep it in warm water for a few minutes. Now close your eyes and place them over it. The tannins in tea will get rid of the puffiness and the lavender will provide moisture. You can also add the tealeaves to warm water and use cotton balls to soak the water up and place over your eyes to soothe puffiness.

After Shave

You can make use of tea bags to soothe shaved skin and also put an end to razor rash. You can add tealeaves to warm water along with some lemon juice and dip cotton balls in it and rub over the rash. If you have a cut then you can skip the lemon and use only the tea. It might sting a little but will help in soothing the eruptions and softening the skin as well. The lemon in it will prevent the skin from tanning.

Shampoo

Tea has the quality of helping in softening the hair. You can use tea to rinse your hair and enhance its softness. If you have dry hair then you can steep 5 tea bags in water and then add in some olive oil to rinse your hair and cleanse it. If you have oily hair then you can steep 5 tea bags in it and add in some lemon juice to rinse your hair. Both of these will work wonders on your hair and nourish it. This will work as both a shampoo and a conditioner for your hair. You can make a batch and use it a couple of times.

Boils

Skin boils can be quite painful and cause an itchy feeling. In order to soothe such boils, you can steep green tea bags in hot water and allow it to release all the flavor. Allow this to cool and then dip cotton balls in it. Now place the ball on the boil and cover it. Keeping this on overnight will help you cut down on the boil and soothe it. You can also steep it in cold water or cool the tea bags and then place them over the boil to enhance its effect.

Hair Color

Don't waste your money on dyes and hair colors, as it is easy for you to color your hair using tea. The tannin will help in turning all your whites into brown. In fact, you can also turn all your blacks into brown as well. All you have to do is heat water and then add in tealeaves and turn it into a brew. Once it cools, you can mix in some beaten egg or fresh yogurt and apply to your head. Allow it to stay for an hour and then wash off with the tea rinse to avail a rich dark color. Doing this regularly can help you get rid of white hair, for good!

Astringent

If you suffer from oily skin, which causes outbursts, then you can make use of tea to solve this problem. You can steep black tea bags in hot water and allow it to moisten. You can then rub the tea bags on your face. You can also dip some cotton balls in it and wipe over your face. This will help you get rid of the oily skin.

Mouth Rinse

In this day and age where everybody is busy leading busy lives, it is obvious that oral hygiene will take a back seat. So, to avail relief from your tooth problems, you can make a simple mouth wash. To make the mouth wash, prepare green tea and then add in some crushed peppermint leaves to it. Allow the leaves to soak in the tea for 10 to 15 minutes and then use it to rinse your mouth. You can also make use of this to avail relief from an aching tooth.

Baby care

Sometimes, babies will keep crying owing to pain from injection. But you can do something to ease the pain and stop your baby from crying. You can steep a tea bag in hot water and place it on the injection site. The tannic acid in it will help soothe your baby's skin and prevent it from stinging.

Tanner

You can use tea to avail a natural tan. The tannin will help in creating an artificial tan. You can steep some regular or black tea bags in hot water and allow the water to go warm. Then, dip cotton balls in it and rub it over your skin. If it is possible to immerse the body part in it then you can do that. This tan can stay with you for quite some time.

Foot Cleanser

Cleansing your feet from time to time will help you maintain clean and hygienic feet. For this, you can steep black tea leaves in hot water and then add in some tea tree oil to it. Allow the two to mix in well and then use it to wash your feet. You can also add it to a bucket of water and lace your feet in it for 10 to 15 minutes. This will help in reducing the odor and also kill any bacteria and other germs. It will aid in cutting down dry feet.

Hand Wash

You can also use tea to make a disinfectant had wash. You can steep green tea bags in hot water and then add in a few tea tree and rose oil drops. Mix it and water to wash your hands. It will help in reducing the germs as also keep your hands soft and moist.

These form the various ways in which you can use tea to prepare cosmetics and toiletries and improve your health and appearance.

Key Highlights

Tea is generally seen as a hot beverage that keeps us awake but what most people don't know is that it is helpful in cleansing the internal organs of the body. It is like washing the body from the inside to get rid of toxins. But you cannot treat it as an elixir that will help you get rid of all the unwanted chemicals in your body. Yes, it is possible to lead a healthier life by drinking tea no doubt but you cannot make it the only thing that will help cleanse your body.

These toxins enter our bodies through various sources and can cause it to slow down. With the use of the right blend of ingredients, it is possible to cleanse the body from the inside out. In fact, it is possible for you to get rid of unwanted elements that circulate in your blood. You will see that these have been eliminated through your urine and sweat. You will feel extremely fit and full of life.

Tea also helps in weight loss. Obesity is now a growing trend and it is important for people to take control. The best way to do so is by consuming teas that are good for the body. The tea contains chemicals that can help in cutting down on the existing fat in your body. It can also help in increasing the digestive power of the body. A chemical known as tannic acid is said to help in these functions.

We looked at the correct ways in which you can prepare the different teas. Many people don't realize that there is a right and a wrong way to prepare teas and simply prepare a tea in general. But you will only be able to savor it fully if you prepare it in the prescribed way. You can go through the list again and learn to prepare tea the best way. As you know, it is best to avoid using tea bags, as their flavor will not be fresh.

There are many things that can affect the quality of tea. Right from the leaf size to the leaf color and the season when the tealeaves are picked, everything will have a bearing on the taste. You can go through the list again and then look for the specific tea leaves to prepare flavorful tea.

We had a look at many recipes and you can prepare and consume them. You don't have to prepare only regular teas and can prepare infusions. You can also prepare food items by making use of teas and tealeaves. These recipes are sure to make you fall in love with the concept of infusing tea in the different savory and sweet dishes. They will help you avail the benefits of teas and you will not have to drink tea for it.

We looked at many myths that surround tea and you have to understand them to savor tea. These myths are mostly based on tea's effectiveness in helping the body remain healthy. Once you go through the list, you will look at the different ways in which tea can help you stay healthy.

As you know, you can make use of tea to prepare cosmetics and toiletries that can help you avail a fit and beautiful body. You have to use the black and green tealeaves and tea bags to prepare these. They are safe and can be used by anyone including children. They will help you save quite a lot of money as they will be cheap to prepare and will also be skin safe. In any case, you might have to test it out on a piece of your skin and see if it is skin friendly.

There are some ingredients that help in controlling your food cravings. At the same time, there are those that help in increasing your appetite. So tea can swing both ways and help you attain good health. You have to identify these teas and savor them based on your needs. Some people consume tea as an appetizer and drink it before having their food. On the other hand, there are some that drink it after a meal to digest the food that they ate.

Remember that the ingredients that you use to prepare these teas need to be as fresh as possible. Try buying them from an organic market near your house. It is also possible for you to grow some of these ingredients at home. All you need is a few pots and seeds that can be planted. You can grow holy basil, fennel and other such herbs. The spices that you use need to be fresh as well as otherwise their flavor can reduce quite a bit.

Although tea is quite safe and anybody can consume, it is important to exercise a little precaution. If you are pregnant or are on medications then it is important to avoid certain herbs and spices. You must consult your doctor before trying out something new. This is especially important for all those that suffer from a condition or take medications on a regular basis. Such people will find it easy to pick the best tea based on their doctor's recommendations.

It is quite easy to make the tea blends at home. All you need is some fresh tealeaves, which you can buy online, and some dried herbs and spices. You can dry the herbs yourself and the spices can be bought online. You can also order a few tea bags, which you can fill with these ingredients and store them in airtight containers. You can create small batches by making use of tea bags. These bags can be used to prepare fresh teas. You can make them and store them for a long time. In general, tea has a long shelf life. You can store them for a year in an airtight container. But do check if it smells good before making use of it.

You can also give your children tea. Just ensure that you tone it down a little. You can give them the ones that are made from fresh herbs. Shankpushpi is especially good for them and will help increase their brainpower.

Conclusion

I thank you once again for choosing this book and hope you had a good time reading it. I'm sure you have now widened your opinion on tea and will look at it from a health point of view. You don't really have to drink an exotic tea on a daily basis and just a regular herbal tea will go a long way in keeping your body strong and healthy.

You can buy the tea infuser and prepare the teas with ease. You must introduce these teas to your friends and family members and help them get their health back on track. Inform them on the importance of avoiding adding milk to their milk and also cut down on the sugar content.

Do not limit yourself to the recipes mentioned in this book and you must experiment and come up with other recipes by yourself. Make use of the ingredients mentioned in this book and use only fresh stuff from organic markets.

Part 2

Introduction

Cleansing is an important process to remove the toxins from your body. Cleansing also known as detoxification can occur naturally to expel waste from your body. The process is necessary because the harmful toxins will not be removed from the body without any external force. There are some chemicals that are used to detoxify your body, but these chemicals can leave poison in your body. You can't take these chemicals without discussing it with your doctor. It will be good to try an alternative, and it can be healthy tea based on natural ingredients.

A cup of green tea based on natural ingredients proves really helpful to flush all toxins from your body. You can drink more than one cup in a day to get rid of body fat and toxins. It has a number of health benefits because you can remove toxins from the body and get a flat belly. If you are following a tea cleanse diet, then it is important to change your eating habits as well. It will lead you to a healthy life because detoxification may help you to avoid a number of diseases. There is a comprehensive diet plan of 14 days that you can follow to get rid of toxins and other dangerous substances of your body.

The 2-week tea cleanse diet is quite safe to boost your metabolism, lose belly fat and flush out toxins. If you want to lose a good amount of weight, then start your diet plan with cleansing. It will help you to shed water weight and make you active. This book is particularly designed for your help so that you can cleanse your body and flush all toxins.

Chapter 1: What Is Cleanse Diet And What Are The Benfefits ?

Detoxification or cleanse diet is a process to remove toxins from the body. This process may involve a number of herbal ingredients, and remedies to cleanse your body. It is important to change your diet and take vitamin supplements. It is the best way to get rid of toxins and enhance the metabolism rate. If you want to detoxify your body, then it is important to follow a particular procedure, such as you need to drink two to three cups of green tea and cut sugar and fat consumption. After following a cleanse diet, there are a number of physical and mental benefits that you can enjoy:

Physical Benefits

The tea cleanses diet will help you to get a number of physical benefits. If you want to remove toxins stored in your organs, then it is important to follow this diet. After detoxification, you will feel lighter and get more energy for other tasks. The detoxification can clear your blood and improve its circulation. It is good for the better health of your immune system. You will be able to enjoy a better health after following this tea cleanse diet.

Increase Your Energy Levels

This 2-week tea cleanse diet will increase your energy because you live on the natural sources of energy like fruits and vegetables. During detox diet, you will reduce sugar intake and live on natural food only. It is important to drink plenty of water during the cleansing program to increase the energy levels.

Remove Additional Waste

The cleanse diet will successfully remove additional waste stored in your body because the purpose of this program is to stimulate your body and help liver, kidneys and colon in their proper functioning.

Proves Helpful in the Weight Loss

With the help of tea cleanse diet, you can shed some pounds, but it will be a short-term weight loss. If you want to lose weight in a healthy way, then it will be good to change your eating habits and follow a healthy diet schedule for a longer period of time. During tea cleanse diet, you drastically reduce the number of calories, but this weight may come back as you replace the good food with unhealthy choices.

Boost Your Immune System

While you are following a tea cleanse diet, you will free your organs from waste and harmful substances. It will give a boost to your immune system and it may be able to absorb good nutrients. You can do a light exercise during tea cleanse diet to reinforce your immunity.

Improve the Health of Your Skin

Skin is the main organ of your body and with tea cleanse diet, you can experience a number of benefits. Sauna during tea cleansing program will help your skin to release excessive toxins. You will get a smooth and clear skin with a detox diet plan.

Improve Your Respiration

This two-week tea cleanse diet will clean your colon because it is a way to release all toxins from your body. It will help you to improve your respiration and get rid of bad breath. It is also good for the digestive system of your body. During detoxification, you may face bad breath, but it will feel better with the passage of time.

Clear Your Mind

This cleansing program will clear your mind and enable you to get rid of stress as well. The cleansing will enhance your ability to think and clear any fog on your senses. Your regular meals are usually stuffed with sugar and fat; therefore, you will feel lethargic. The cleanse diet will clear the fog from your mind, and you may be able to take better decisions with fresh mind.

Beautiful Hair

If you are worried about your dead hair, then try this cleanse diet to stimulate the growth of hair follicles. After detoxification of your body, you will clearly see the difference in your hair. It will make them shiny, silky and soft, and you may experience rapid growth of hair.

Anti-aging and Cleansing

Toxins in your body can trigger the aging process; therefore, it is important to remove the amount of radicals in your body. These will increase your age and reduce the speed of the aging process. If you want to enjoy its long-term benefits, then it will be good to make a permanent change in your lifestyle after detoxification. The 2-week tea cleanse diet can improve your health and you will feel even lighter than before.

Chapter 2: Healthy Natural Teas To Cleanse Your Body

There are numerous health benefits of tea cleanse diet because it enables you to reduce weight quickly and clean your colon. The tea cleanses diet will put your body in hunger mode, and this practice is quite old to clean your body and colon. There are several varieties of teas that you can use to clean your kidneys, liver, and colon. You should restrict to fruits, vegetables, broths and herbal teas to clean your digestive system. This diet will last for 14 days to completely cleanse your body.

Types of Teas that You can Use

There are a number of varieties that you can try to cleanse your body, including senna tea, ginseng tea, green tea, and various other teas. Senna tea is good for its laxative and diuretic properties because it can lose weight by expelling out fecal materials and water from your body. Green tea is perfect to use in the detox diet to burn fat and increase your metabolism. You can also prepare a green tea with a combination of Guarana, bitter orange, kelp, and ginseng. This tea will reduce your hunger and remove toxic elements from your body.

How do you shed some pounds?

With the help of tea cleanse diet; you can experience a dramatic reduction in the weight. You can shed almost 20 pounds in two weeks because this process expels water and waste material out of your body. This weight loss will be proved to temporary weight loss as you return to your normal diet; therefore, it is recommended to include natural food items in your diet. During this diet, you need to consume almost 500 or fewer calories on a regular basis. In this way, you are giving a deficit of 1 pound in the weight after every two to three days.

Types of Herbal Teas for Detoxification

You can make green tea for detoxification at home to improve your overall health. The Green tea is perfect to use during this process, but if you get bored of the similar taste of green tea on a regular basis, then you can try this below given recipe to change your mood:

Green Smooth Tea With Apple

If you want to get the benefits of green smoothies, then try this green tea easy to do with lots of nutrition. To make this you will need:

- 1 cup brewed Green Tea

- ½ Apple

- ½ cup Baby Kale

- 1 Tablespoon Fat-Free Yogurt

- Ice (Optional)

Instructions:

Make a blend of all these components to get a smooth mixture. If you want to load it with additional fiber, then use avocado. You can't skip Green Tea because it is an important part of this mixture.

3 P Juice And Green Tea

You can prepare a blend of pineapple, papaya and pear because these are loaded with Vitamin C to detoxify your body. It will load your cup with fiber as well, so make the juice of three powerful fruits and mix it with a cup of green tea. It will be a special drink for the health of your immune system. To make this blend, you will need:

- 1 cup green tea

- ½ pear

- ½ cup of pineapple

- ½ cup of papaya

Procedure:

Cut the fruits into small slices and then blend them to make juice. You need to blend thoroughly to get a smooth blend. It will make your green tea really yummy and interesting.

Wake Up Shake

You will naturally get caffeine through a cup of Gren tea and it is enough to start your morning without a headache. It is a delicious way to send a message to the body and brain that it is time to wake up and move on. To make it, you will need:

- 1 teaspoon Green Tea Powder

- ½ orange without seeds

- 1/4 grapefruit without seeds

- ½ Banana

- 1 cup coconut milk

- 1 cup ice

Procedure:

Make a smooth blend of all ingredients in a blender with protein powder for additional taste. Enjoy this yummy cup of green tea for your lunch as well because it can increase your satisfaction for longer times.

Green Tea Frappe

Are you looking for a fancy beverage just like the one you can get in a coffee shop? Add green tea matcha powder in the drink and give it a unique taste. This type of powerful beverage is used in the Japanese ceremonies with a unique flavor. It has a number of health benefits for you. In order to make this tea, you should have:

- 1 Teaspoon Green Tea Matcha Powder

- I cup fresh coconut milk

- 1 cup ice

Procedure:

Make a smooth blend of all the ingredients to get a creamy and foamy texture. This cool drink will be an idea for the summer season. It will make you full and enhance your metabolism.

Tropical Green Smoothie

You can use a number of tropical fruits to enhance the taste of this green drink. The Mango, Papaya, Banana, and coconut milk will give you an excellent mixture.

These fruits are full of fiber, potassium, and antioxidants. These are good to enhance the power of your immune system:

Things You Need:

- 1 teaspoon Matcha Powder

- ½ cup papaya in the forms of cubes

- ½ cup of fresh mango

- ½ Banana

- ½ cup papaya

- 1 cup coconut milk

- 1 cup ice

Procedure:

Put all ingredients in the blender to make a blend. You can add or remove an ingredient from the recipe to enhance its taste. It will be a smooth mixture for every season because you can change the fruits with the available options in the market.

Spicy Green Tonic

The green tea can be mixed with spices to enjoy a number of health benefits. Make a cup of tonic mixed with spices to provide essential nutrients to your body. Turmeric and cinnamon have loads of anti-inflammatory and antioxidants. You will need various things, such as:

- 1 big cup of hot water for Green Tea

- ¼ teaspoon of Turmeric

- 1/7 Teaspoon of Cinnamon

- 8 ounces of purified water at boiling point

Procedure:

Take a tea bag and spices and pour into a hot water you have prepared for your tea. You can use different spices to make a blend, such as cayenne pepper. It is good to improve your metabolism. The ginseng or ginger is equally good to cleanse your body. You can use different spices like basil, rosemary, cumin, nutmeg, saffron, cardamom, curry, thyme, etc.

Energy Boosting Smoothie

If you are feeling dull, then it is time to store energy and this smoothie will help you. Just buy blueberries, raspberries and yogurt make this energized drink. You will need:

- Cup green tea

- ¼ cup clean raspberries

- ¼ cup clean blueberries

- 1 teaspoon fat-free yogurt

- 1 cup of ice

Procedure:

Just make a blend of all ingredients and try this to lose weight. The frozen berries can also be used, but it will be good to try fresh. You should take it in the morning to enhance your energy.

Chapter 3: 2 Week Tea Cleanse Diet Plan

There are most likely times where your body will feel lethargic, rundown and drowsy. On the off chance that that is the situation, you either need to get more rest, or you have to detox. There are a lot of approaches to detox, yet the simplest form is by detoxing with herbs. Detoxing will assist clean with excursion your inner parts and uproot poisons and overabundance liquids that have attacked your body and stolen your vitality. In addition, it will advantage your hair, skin and nails and assist you with sleeping better.

The most difficult part about following a diet is always the DIET PLAN!! Figuring out what to eat and when to eat is probably the biggest reason as to why people fail at successfully accomplishing this goal. Getting recipes and then cooking that particular food when everyone else is eating those delicious burgers can be really hard. Well, we can't really help you with the cooking part but we sure can help you provide a routine to follow for 2 weeks and some recipes that are not only delicious but are healthy as well.

For the detox you will be eating a fluid meal, for example, a shake for breakfast and a solid supper from the Detox Diet for lunch and dinner. This diet plan is only a proposal. We included heaps of diverse recipes to outline all the astonishing alternatives out there. In the event that it is excessively overpowering feel free to substitute simpler meals or bigger portions to eat for a few days. But eat CLEAN.2-week tea cleanse diet will help you to flush out toxins and get a healthy body. Following is a simple diet plan for your guidance.

Day One

For the first day, at around 7 am or whenever you wake up; drink a glass of room temperature lemon water. Although this is not as appetizing but warm lemon water in the morning helps kickstart the digestion process for the day.

Step By Step Instruction

You should use filtered water and it ought to be warm not very hot. You should avoid ice cold water, since that can be a harder for your body to process and it takes more vitality to process super cold water than the warm. Continuously utilize new lemons, organic if conceivable, never packaged lemon juice. Press 1/2 a lemon with every glass and drink it down first thing before you eat anything or workout. You can always add freshly grated ginger.

Around 8 am drink 1 cup of herbal tea. You can choose from a variety of herbal teas and it is not important to drink the same tea every day. For example, you can drink Cinnamon Tea. This will help you boost your memory and concertation.

For 1.25 Cup

1. Place 1.5 mugs water into pot or glass pot

2. Add one Ceylon Cinnamon Stick (3-inch length)

3. Slowly boil the Cinnamon sticks to extract the flavor properly. Boil the cinnamon sticks for about 15-20 minutes at low-medium heat. Bubbling quick won't blend the Cinnamon appropriately. You will note even after the water has gone to a full heat up, the water's shade is still just a light yellow.

4. Once the water starts bubbling let the sticks cool for 15 minutes.

5. After the cinnamon discharges, strain the tea through a fine strainer and drink it.

For breakfast, at around 10 am have

Chai Gingerbread Shake

Ingredients

- 1 teaspoon cinnamon

- 1 cup warm brewed rooibos chai tea

- 2 teaspoons ground ginger

- 1/2 teaspoon allspice

- raw honey to taste

- 1/2 cup coconut milk

- 1 scoop protein powder

Method

Mix until smooth. Drink before it cools.

At 11.30am have another mug of hot lemon water or herbal tea.

For lunch, there is a variety of option. You can have Chickpea Soup for example.

At 4 pm, you can consume a snack. Walnut Lentil Pate is an example of the snack you can eat. The will have an early dinner which is around 6 pm. You can have Quinoa Stuffed Kabocha.

Day Two

Similarly to the first, you are going to drink a glass of warm water with lemon in it. Then around 8 am pick an herbal tea; for example Goji Berry. It is still moderately unprecedented today, however, considered a staple of old Chinese medication, the goji berry is thought to have advantages to both the liver and kidneys, subsequently its incorporation in numerous detoxification regimens.

For breakfast at around 10 am you can have a peppermint hot chocolate. The main idea for breakfast is to have liquid shakes and smoothies in cooperating plants and other whole foods.

Ingredients

- 1/4 cup sugar

- 1 1/2 cup heavy cream

- 1/8 teaspoon salt

- 1 1/2 cups milk

- 6 ounces bittersweet chocolate, chopped

- Sweetened whipped cream, for garnish

- 3 drops peppermint oil

- Chocolate shavings, for garnish

Method

In a pot, combine the cream, sugar, milk, and salt and warm over medium-low warmth. At the point when the cream blend just starts to steam, include the cleaved chocolate, and mix, until softened. Blend in the peppermint oil. Isolate the hot chocolate among mugs and top with whipped cream and chocolate shaving.

At 11.30, intake a hot mug of lemon water or herbal tea. Lemon water contains Vitamin C which is our immune system booster. The level of vitamin C in your framework is one of the first things to fall when you're focused on, which is the reason specialists suggested popping additional vitamin C amid particularly unpleasant days.The delicious roasted and clean carrot soup can be had for lunch at 1.30 pm. At 4 pm, you can have a handful of mixed seeds and or almonds. This will not only reduce any cravings but will also give you added benefits. Pan Chicken and Broccoli is appetizing and also fulfilling. Have that for dinner at 6 pm.

Day Three

So we will repeat the same drill for the third day as well starting with a glass of room temperature with lemon in it. In the event that you drink lemon water all the time, it will diminish the acidity in your body, which is the place illness states happen. It eliminates uric acid in your joints, which is one of the fundamental drivers of inflammation.

In addition, lemon water improves heart health, brain, and nerve function since it is high in potassium. Developing a habit of drinking lemon water daily will ONLY benefit you since it has numerous advantages.

Around 8 am have herbal tea. For instance, you can have spearmint tea. Peppermint is unbelievably common in the natural tea world both because of its heavenly flavor and known medical advantages. Be that as it may, its relative spearmint is just as vital because of its contained cell reinforcements and capacity to fight off common health problems like tummy inconveniences.

Ingredients

- A kettleful of filtered water (about 2 to 4 cups depending on how strong you want your)

- a handful of fresh mint leaves

- Honey to taste

Method

1. Roughly tear the leaves with your hands and spot them in a little strainer set over a teapot or glass dish.

2. Bring the water to a bubble and pour over the clears out. (The water ought to cover the leaves in the strainer)

3. Gently press the mint leaves with the back of a wooden spoon or a muddler to discharge the oils.

4. Cover the teapot or bowl and let the leaves steep for no less than 5 to 10 minutes, then evacuate the strainer pushing on the leaves to concentrate however much fluid as could reasonably be expected.

5. Pour into tea mugs or mug and sweeten with nectar or sugar to taste if craved.

At around 10 am have Savory Shake for your breakfast.

Kale And Apple Green Smoothie

Ingredients

- ⅔ cup almond milk (unsweetened)

- 1 ½ cups kale (chopped, packed)

- ¾ cup ice

- ½ Gala apple (cut into chunks)

- 1 stalk celery (diced)

- Agave nectar (to taste)

- 1 tbsp ground flax seed

  Method

- Combine almond milk, kale, ice, apple, celery, and flax seed in a blender. Blend on high until smooth.

- Taste smoothie. Add agave nectar if needed and blend again.

At 11.30 have a mug of lemon water or herbal tea.

Honeybush is enjoyed consistently as a cancer prevention agent tea and is appreciated routinely due to its heavenly flavor. It needs caffeine and is likewise brimming with sound vitamins like vitamin C, calcium, magnesium and potassium, all supplements the body needs to capacity at its crest.

Ingredients

- 3 parts Honeybush

- 1 part Lavender

- The juice of 1/2 lemon or orange

- 1 part Rooibos (optional)

- 1 part Oatstraw

Method

Combine all. Steep 1 tablespoon in 16 ounces boiled water for 6 minutes. Strain and enjoy!

For lunch have the delicious Balsamic Miso Root Salad. The best part about having salads is that you can consume it even in larger portions. At 4 pm have some Walnut Lentil Pate. This will aid with the feeling of deprivation. If you feel less deprived you would intake less food. At 6 pm, have the final meal of the day. You can have coconut poached salmon.

So this was a simple sample diet plan. This is a very good example of a 2 week cleanse diet plan. This is because it adds lemon water twice a day. By know, I believe you a clear on how important lemon water is for our health as it aids in digestion and protects from major and minor health issues. Furthermore, it adds herbal tea. There are a gazillion options when it comes to choosing the herbal tea; each one having its own benefits. The best thing about this diet is that you can either have the same herbal tea throughout the 2 weeks or you can try out all the different kinds.

For breakfast, you are supposed to have a shake using plant based proteins and whole foods. For lunch, you are required to have a solid meal which is approved by the detox diet food list. Your main focus should be on vegetables, healthy fats and lean proteins. There is a mouthwatering snack included in the diet to fulfill any evening cravings.The dinner must be light, largely focusing on soup, salad and vegetables. Follow this pattern for two weeks and you will find yourself full of energy and healthy as ever.Hopefully, you have understood the sample of the kind of diet that you should follow when on a tea cleanse diet.

Two Week Rapid Weight Loss Plan

Everybody just wants to lose weight fast these days; this is why we would suggest this two-week rapid weight loss plan. This diet plan will not only shed pounds but also decrease the diseases. Diseases such as type 2 diabetes, symptoms of food sensitivity, and chronic pain begins to dissipate with this diet.

What can you eat?

Lemon Water: When you wake up drink a glass of hot water with half a lemon. This beverage is going to kick start your digestive procedure for the day. Old societies have trusted that lemon helps weight reduction by purging the liver.

Breakfast Smoothie—You need to eat—right? I need you to have a breakfast smoothie pressed with protein to keep you full for a considerable length of time. The following recipe makes a quick and easy smoothie that contains cancer prevention agents that will scrub you of poisons and support your immunity:

Ingredients

- 2 tablespoons of rice protein powder

- ½ banana

- 1 cup of unsweetened almond milk

- ½ cup of frozen berries

- 2 tablespoons of flaxseed powder

Mix well in the blender and enjoy your smoothie!

Green Tea: It is a great antioxidant drink. For this diet, opt for a green tea that is organic. Green tea can be used to replace the coffee and add fat-burning catechism compounds.

Proteins: You can have 6 ounces of protein consisting of turkey, chicken or fish—to help keep you full. This way you will not feel drained or get a sense of deprivation.

Carbs: The idea is to avoid starches. But simply put, we do not want to be cruel so you can consume half cup of brown rice per day. Otherwise, you cannot take any carbs.

Fats: The intake of good fats in moderation is allowed. Olive oil and avocado are examples of good fats.Olive oil and avocado contain healthy types of fats that your body needs.

Dairy: Greek yogurt has calcium in it that will help melt fat. This is why only 1 cup of 2% Greek yogurt is allowed. Other than that no dairy products are allowed on this 2-week diet plan.

Vegetables: You can have the unlimited amount of low GI vegetables and Detox broth.

Snacks consisting of hummus, nuts and/or pickles—a couple of handfuls a day are allowed.

You can have any of these once a day, whenever you feel like it, which means there is no time restriction on this.

What You Need To Eliminate.

1. Wheat—this is as a matter of fact is the hardest part of the entire diet — we request you that you wipe out the wheat from your eating regimen. Eliminating wheat does not only helps in reducing weight, but it also determines what goes to the brain as well. A number of people suffer from gluten sensitivities and what happens is that the gluten found in wheat, sugars, and different wellsprings of starches are bringing about an inflammation that is deceiving the cerebrum into craving even more food. Although, 1/2 cup of brown rice is acceptable once a day.

2. Artificial Sweeteners—eliminating artificial sweeteners is also crucial. To be clear, this is all the diet soft drinks you all are depending on, and the blue, pink and yellow packets that people are getting off the table, which are basically all the artificial sweeteners utilized for adding to espresso and tea when at an eatery or at home. Studies demonstrate that utilizing simulated sweeteners adds 70% more to your waist size.Stevia is a magnificent, zero calories, all normal sweeteners to consider if your food and beverages taste a bit insipid. If you utilize sweeteners routinely you may have an unpleasant time kicking the enslavement. Give it 4 days prior to the longings vanish. When you lose the yearnings you will have practically zero longing to re-bring them into your eating routine.

3. Refined Sugar and Alcohol—Be that as it may, wiping out artificial sweeteners likewise incorporates disposing of refined table sugar to those sugars found in liquor. In spite of the fact that this is the hardest part for some individuals to stick to, what you need to understand is that the craving is only temporary.The first day or two after you move beyond the addictive piece of the nourishment you are eating, it's [the sugar craving] kind of eases up. Eventually, you understand the importance of eating healthy.

4. Coffee—Here's the reason why it is imperative to dispense coffee from this diet plan —most of you don't drink espresso dark, so you add sugar and cream to it, which are void calories and empty fat. Likewise, coffee winds up being a trigger for the most of you. It's a trigger that makes you eat a considerable measure of the nourishments that joins it like the donut in the morning or the cake. The other thing is that you drink a lot of espressos and it lifts your cortisol, which gives you a misguided feeling of energy. Furthermore, it disturbs your hormones that in turn bring about expanded eating and your weight increases.

5. Dairy—Dairy is the foundation of a lot of food sensitivities that causes aggravation in your body, and it is advised that you have Greek yogurt instead.

Other Things To Do

Take Probiotics and Nutrients

The last step is adding probiotics and supplements to accelerate the weight reduction. A probiotic is important in light of the fact that it energizes the great microorganisms in your digestion tracts. You will likewise need to have a multivitamin in the event of some unforeseen issue, in light of the fact that a great deal of you were going from a system where you weren't eating the right things.

Take a multivitamin

A multivitamin will accelerate the weight reduction process and, in addition, give our bodies the supplements that we have to work more ready and fiery. Also, a quality multivitamin will keep our resistant immune systems healthier and advance bone quality, heart wellbeing, skin wellbeing and general prosperity. A body rich in supplements and vitamins will release the fat effortlessly assisting you with seeing results sooner.

(Take a probiotic each morning and 1/2 of a multivitamin in the morning and a half at night)

Detox Bath

Take a detox bath every night. In order to do so add 1 cup of baking soda and soak with 2 cups of Epsom salt.

Low GI-Vegetables

In order to quickly lose weight, you should add Unlimited Quantities of Low Glycemic Food to Burn Fat Fast.Our bodies store glycogen from the sugars we allow.

These low-glycemic lists of veggies kick begin our bodies into blazing off the abundance glycogen. As our glycogen levels diminish the weight begins to tumble off when these vegetables are brought into our eating methodologies.

These are only a portion of the delightful low-glycemic file veggies that you can eat as much as you need to. You can likewise present a low sodium vegetable stock and add these veggies to make a tasty soup!

- Artichoke

- Artichoke hearts

- Asparagus

- Bamboo shoots

- Bean sprouts

- Brussel Sprouts

- Broccoli

- Cauliflower

- Celery

- Cucumber

- Daikon

- Eggplant

- Leeks

- Lentils

- Beans (green, kidney, garbanzo)

- Greens (collard, kale, mustard, turnip)

- Mushrooms

- Okra

- Onions

- Pea pads

- Peppers

- Radishes

- Squash

- Sugar snap peas

- Swiss chard

- Tomato

- Water chestnuts

- Watercress

- Zucchini

- Cabbage (green, bok choy, Chinese)

- Salad greens(chicory, endive, escarole, iceberg lettuce, romaine, spinach, arugula, radicchio, watercress)

Shopping List

- Baking soda

- Green tea

- 1 bottle olive oil

- Epsom salt

- Balsamic vinegar (or any other vinegar for salad dressing)

- Rice protein powder (28 tablespoons)

- One and three-fourth cups of ground flaxseeds

- Three and a half cups of brown rice

Shopping List (Each Week Buy)

- 4 bananas

- 4 lemons

- 2 qts unsweetened vanilla almond milk

- 56 oz froze berries

- 4 avocados

- 7 plain 2% Greek yogurts (6-oz serving size)

- One and a half pounds of chicken, turkey or fish combined

- Shopping List (Detox Vegetable Broth)

- 4 cups root vegetable (any of the following: turnips, parsnips, rutabagas)

- 8 cups chopped greens (any of the following: kale, parsley, beef greens, collard greens, chard, and dandelion)

- 8 carrots

- 8 celery stalks

- Dried ginger

- 4 large onions

- 4 cups winter squash

- 2 cups cabbage

- 8 cloves whole garlic

The Top 10 Tea And Smoothie Recipes

All-About-The-Berries Smoothie

Berries are your companion in the matter of detoxing on account of the considerable number of cell reinforcements and fiber they contain. They're only the thing your body needs to renew itself and to help cleanse poisons from its different frameworks. Blueberries are stuffed with them, and raspberries and blackberries likewise have a ton, so we'll utilize every one of the three here to verify it's a detox champ.

Ingredients

- 1/2 containers Berry Mix (Blueberries, Raspberries, Blackberries)

- 1/8 container moved oats

- 1 container Purified Water

- 1/2 container Coconut Milk

Method

Blend everything together until you achieve a smoothie consistency. The excellence of berries is their simple prep. New berries require a wash before going in while solidified you simply pop right in. At the point when detoxing natural produce is constantly suggested.

Cocoa Bliss Smoothie

You can utilize chocolate as a component of your detox schedule, insofar as it's the right kind. This smoothie poses a flavor like chocolate covered strawberries, sweet and chocolatey with digestive proteins from the nectar, no refined sugar, and cell reinforcements from the chocolate and strawberries.

Ingredients

- 1 tbsp Dark Cocoa Powder

- 1/2 cup Strawberries

- 1/2 cup Coconut Milk

- 1 cup Ice

Blend everything together until frothy and smooth.

Cashew Cream Smoothie
Ingredients

- 1 cup coconut water OR nut/rice/hemp seed milk of your choice

- 1 handful cashews

- 1 ripe mango pitted and diced

- 2 handfuls mixed berries (fresh or frozen: blackberries, blueberries, raspberries)

- 2 heaping tablespoons plant-based protein powder (ideally vanilla flavor)

- optional: 1 tablespoon ground flax seed

    Method

It's really simple to make, just blend all the ingredients until they are creamy and then add a pinch of salt.

The Grasshopper Shake

Ingredients

- 1 heaping tablespoon cacao powder

- 1½ cups warm peppermint tea

- 2 tablespoon whole cashews

- 1 tablespoon melted coconut oil

- ¼ teaspoon stevia

- 2 teaspoons spirulina (you can use chlorella or any green powder)

- pinch of sea salt

These are optional ingredients, just to add a little more flavor:

- 2 heaping tablespoons plant-based protein powder (ideally chocolate flavor)

- optional: 1 tablespoon ground flax seed

Method

Pour the warm tea into a blender. Include cacao powder, cashews, spirulina, salt and stevia and mix for 45 seconds or until cashews are separated. While blending, sprinkle in the liquefied coconut oil. Serve in a mug for a nutritious and warm drink.

Sexy Cilantro Shake

Ingredients

- 1 cup coconut water

- 1 cup rice/nut/seed milk

- 3 dates OR stevia to taste

- 1 cup fresh cilantro leaves

- 1 cup papaya (fresh), peeled and diced

- ½ cup fresh or frozen mango or peaches

Method

Mix all ingredients together until smooth. It's been demonstrated that cilantro is extraordinarily detoxifying and can assist pull metal from the body, so drink up, particularly in the event that you live in a city, have mercury fillings, or beverage faucet water!

Peach Apple Cobbler

Ingredients

- 1 cup was frozen or fresh peaches

- ¼ cup pecans (whole or crushed)

- 1 tablespoon fresh lemon juice

- 1 cup coconut water

- 1 teaspoon cinnamon

- 2 apples (any variety), cored and sliced into chunks (if organic, leave the peel on for added fiber and nutrients)

- ½ teaspoon ginger powder

- 2 teaspoons vanilla powder or extract

- Pinch of sea salt

Blend all ingredients together until creamy and enjoy!

Chocolate Covered Blueberries

Ingredients

- 1 handful of spinach

- dash of cinnamon

- 1 large handful of frozen blueberries

- 2 tablespoons almond butter

- 1 tablespoon of raw cacao

- ½ coconut milk and ½ coconut water (as much as you need for your blender) or you could replace the coconut water with green tea.

- 2 heaping tablespoons plant-based protein powder (ideally chocolate flavor)

- dash of stevia as needed

- optional: 1 tablespoon ground flax seed

Blend and enjoy!

Sweet Protein Shake

Ingredients

- 1 cup nuts (pecans, walnuts, or almonds)

- 5-10 drops stevia extract (to taste)

- Your choice of rice/almond/hemp seed milk (just enough to cover nuts in the base of the blender)

- 1 teaspoon vanilla extract

- 1 apple

- 2-3 cups froze fruit (blueberries, raspberries, blackberries, mangoes, papaya, peaches)

- 1 ripe pear

- Water OR brewed and cooled herbal tea (like ginger, raspberry, lemon, rooibos, green, yerba mate, etc.)

- OR coconut water (just enough to blend to desired consistency)

- 2 heaping tablespoons plant-based protein powder

- optional: 1 tablespoon ground flax seed

Blend all ingredients until smooth.

Keepin' It Smooth

Ingredients

- 1 avocado

- 1 handful of raspberries

- 5 ounces frozen peaches

- unsweetened almond milk

- 1 handful of hemp seeds

- 2 heaping tablespoons plant-based protein powder

- 2 dates

- this ingredient is optional: 1 tablespoon ground flax seed

Blend and Enjoy!

Green And Clean Smoothie

This smoothie is straight out of a Sesame Street scene in light of the fact that we're simply going to concentrate on green things. Open your cooler and haul out anything green, odds are it's a sound vegetable alternative. You can likewise lift these up from the store whenever you're out on the off chance that you need to take after along splendidly.

Ingredients

- 1/4 Cucumber

- 1/2 Avocado

- 1/2 modest bunch Spinach or Other Leafy Green

- 2 sprigs Fresh Mint

- 1 Celery stalk

- 1 glass Purified Water

- 1 Kiwifruit

- Squirt of lemon

- 1/2 of apple

Blend everything together in your blender. In case you're utilizing natural cucumber (suggested) you can leave the peels on for included dietary worth.

Chapter 4: Useful Herbs To Use During Cleanse Diet

Cleaning is not only important for your home, but for your body because it will help you to get rid of harmful chemicals. In the winter, summer and spring, you can detoxify your body. The use of herbal tea will be a great start to getting your body cleansed. There are numerous detox herbs that you can include in your diet. It will support your liver, kidneys and other organs of the body. Following are some good herbs to include in your cleanse diet:

Dandelion

It is a famous detox herb to cleanse your liver and promote the production of bile. It enables your body to remove toxins. You can add a few leaves of Dandelion in a salad or make a tea with its roots.

Milk Thistle

This is an active herb to avoid liver damage and generate new cells frequently. You can use silymarin, an active part of milk thistle in the form of a capsule. You can use it with a concentrated supplement because it is not soluble in the body with water. A 200 mg capsule is good for you in a day.

Turmeric

It is an excellent herb for the liver to stimulate the bile flow and remove the toxins from the whole body. A 50mg turmeric supplement is good for you to include in your diet. You can also add it in your food items.

Green Tea

Keep it in mind that the body cleansing is incomplete without green tea because it helps you to cleanse your body and fight with cancer cells. It can protect your body from a number of chemicals and toxins that can cause cancer. Try to drink two cups of green tea in a day.

Garlic

It has sulfur compounds to oxidize heavy metals in your body and increase their solubility in water. You can remove these compounds easily with the use of water. The garlic can improve the strength of your immune system and control the flow of free radicals. You can eat raw garlic in crushed form.

Cilantro

It is good to reduce cadmium, aluminum, mercury and make it easy for your body to expel them out. You can make a cup of cilantro green tea and take ¼ cup once in a day for three weeks.

Natural Gum Acacia

The sap of the acacia tree is helpful to relieve diarrhea and improve bowel movements. You can use it to improve electrolyte inclusion. It is famous for its oxypower and you can make a blend of this herb by mixing it with hydrocolloid.

Black Walnut

It was introduced in Europe in 1600's and can be used to get rid of harmful bacteria in your body. You have to use it to reduce the harmful elements from body organs and increase their lifespan.

Alfalfa Leaf

These are famous leaves used for the treatment of various infections. You can use them for stomach ulcers and treat your hunger problems. It can be helpful to remove lots of bad elements from your body.

Peppermint

It is commonly found in your kitchen and it is commonly used for cold and flu. You can use this herb for the treatment of sinus infection and sore throat. It will increase the immunity of your body and cleanse your lungs.

Eucalyptus

If you want to cleanse your lungs, then try this diet because it enables you to fight with bacterial and virus attacks. It is good for chest congestion and perfect for its soothing properties.

Stinging Nettle for Blood Pressure

The antioxidant properties of this herb can increase your resistance to inflammation and reduce your blood pressure to a normal level.

Chapter 5: Things To Completely Avoid During Two-Week Tea Cleanse Diet

If you want to make your two-week tea cleanse diet successfully, then it is important to completely avoid these items:

- Dairy, eggs, butter, and mayonnaise are not allowed in any conditioned during cleanse diet. You can't take any kind of these food items.

- Completely remove grains from your diet like wheat, spelled, rye, oats, Kamut, triticale, etc.

- Some fruits and vegetables like creamy vegetables, oranges, and orange juices are not allowed to use.

- There is no need to take canned meat, shellfish, frankfurters, pork, beef, veal and cold cuts.

- Soybean products like the soy yogurt, milk, tofu, and beans are not good to take during body cleanse diet.

- Peanuts, seeds, peanut butter and other similar items should not be taken.

- There is no need to take processed oils, salad dressings, cheese, spreads, etc.

- Alcohol, soft drinks, and caffeinated drinks are completely banned during tea cleanse diet.

- Rice and sugar, either brown or white should not be taken during this diet. You have to avoid all sugars, honey, artificial sweeteners, corn syrup, and cane juices.

- Say no to chocolate, ketchup, sauces, teriyaki and relishes during the tea cleaning diet process.

- Control your salt intake because the sodium may promote water retention in your body.

By avoiding all these food items, you can get considerable benefits of this diet.

Common Mistakes to Avoid During Tea Cleanse Diet

The 2-week tea cleanse diet is really beneficial for you, but there are some mistakes that can ruin your diet. You should avoid these mistakes:

Depriving Your Body

The basic purpose of tea cleanse diet is to nourish your body with essential nutrients. You are supposed to eat fresh fruits and vegetables instead of starving yourself. The deprivation may lead you to low energy, nausea, stress, headaches, irritation, joint aches, and tension. You need to provide essential vitamins, minerals and nutrients to your body. Make sure to provide enough fiber to your body to eliminate toxins. The fiber will glue the toxins in your body and escort them out forcefully.

Quick Cleansing

You spend a major part of your life in a toxic environment, and you are supposed to remove toxins from your body in a few days. It is not wise because quick cleansing will promote weight gain instead of weight loss. Your body can eliminate toxins at once, and after one-time cleansing, your body may become overwhelmed. If you do it repeatedly, then you may bear nausea, headaches or various other problems. A 14 to 30-day detox program is good to boost weight loss and reduce side effects.

Start Cleansing Without Making Your Mind

If you want to detoxify your body, it is important to start with your mind because with the change in thoughts, you will feel better. You have to get rid of your toxic thoughts and change your lifestyle to adjust these changes in your life. It will be good to involve your body in a physical activity to get rid of toxins.

Dehydration

While following the two-week tea cleanse diet, it is important to drink plenty of water. People often fail to drink enough water and it may lead them to dehydration. If you want to expel toxins of your body out, it is essential to drink plenty of water on a regular basis. Start your day with a three to four glasses of water with lemon followed by green tea. Make sure to add lemon in your water to promote fat loss.

Tips to Retain Weight Lost During Tea Cleanse Diet

It is true that the weight that you will decrease with tea cleanse diet can come back once you resume your normal diet. Fortunately, it is possible to retain this weight for a longer period of time. After tea cleanse diet, it is not good to move instantly to your normal diet. Keep an eye on your eating habits, and try to include vegetables and fruits in your regular diet. Instead of consuming wheat, have a healthy substitute available in the form of oats.

You can prefer brown rice instead of white rice and cut the consumption of white sugar. It will be good to fulfill the sugar needs of your body via natural fruits. Go for a brisk walk five times a week and try to involve your body in regular exercise. Try to use stairs instead of the lift and prefer to travel on foot for short distances. It will not only help you to maintain your lost weight but may shed a few more pounds. You have to drink plenty of water because 12 to 14 glasses of water are necessary to drink on a regular basis. It will keep you hydrated and improve the speed of your metabolism.

After following this diet plan, you will surely reduce a good amount of weight and retain it for a longer period of time. It would be better to wait for at least two to three months to repeat this tea cleanse diet to maintain your health because excessive cleansing may lead you to various drawbacks like a headache, irritation, and deprivation. It is safe to repeat it almost after three months to expel harmful toxins out of your body. If you want to stay healthy and fit forever, then it will be good to do friendship with fresh fruits and vegetables.

Chapter 6: Benefits Of A Tea Cleanse

Unlike other detoxes, the tea cleanse is one of the easiest to follow. But that is not a valid reason for anyone to opt for it; even if you are convinced that you have lots of toxins in your body than anyone else.

Before we go on to look at the benefits of the tea detox, we must make one thing clear. Taking a cleanse doesn't mean that your body is no longer capable of cleaning itself. The point is to give it a little push as we now consume more toxins than our previous generations.

Just take a look your plate! It is probably filled with unhealthy food.

Here are some of the reason you may need to do a tea cleanse:

Increased Energy

Your digestive system is like a computer. If you use it without cleaning, dust will collect inside and block the air vents. So it will not operate efficiently. You will notice that it is overheating and even shutting down in the waste scenarios.

If you can see your body in the same way, you will not have a hard time understanding the benefits of a tea cleanse. With years of eating junk, your digestive system will become glacial. It will be unfit to carry out its duties, and as a result, you start to feel weak.

But if you detox, you will remove all the waste that has gathered in your digestive system. The body will be able to digest and absorb food properly.

You Will Lose Weight

Did you break the scale the last time you were on it? Blame it on bad food. Have you had to buy new clothes because the old ones don't fit anymore? Blame it on bad food too. And if your dog is misbehaving, he hasn't seen an alien. It's probably because of bad food.
Current diets are not ideal for healthy living, let alone maintaining a healthy weight.
Much of our food is high in calories, and at the same time, we eat more than we need.
But if you can take the tea cleanse, you will give your body a break from the junk. This will help it clean itself.
The tea cleanse promotes eating healthy food that is also low in calories.

Improved Immunity

We all have dangerous organisms in our bodies. And if these are given freedom to prevail, they can destroy us. Unfortunately, having all kinds of toxins is a surefire way to provide a breeding ground for these organisms.
Thankfully for you, you have the tea cleanse. If only you can take it, you would be able to remove all these dangerous organisms from your body.
With your body cleaned, diseases won't attack you easily. Additionally, since the tea detox will result in the

absorption of more nutrients, you will boost your immunity.

Promotes Healthy Skin

The skin is the largest organ in the body. It has a total area of 20 square feet. Apart from that, it's also very crucial in the removal of wastes from the body.

But with time, it can get clogged with toxins. So it may start to struggle in removing wastes. And this has negative effects on your body.

With a tea detox, however, you can turn things around. You can flush out any toxins gathering under the skin.

In the end, not only will your skin work efficiently, but it will also look healthy, which is a bonus if you spend money on beauty products.

Reduces the Effects of Smoking

1 in every 3 people smoke. And that's a lot if you consider the dangers of smoking. Many claim they do this to reduce stress (possibly, after a fight with the significant other). For others, it's just an addiction.

Smoking is very dangerous. And among those dangers is the increased risk of lung cancer.

With a tea detox, you can reverse some of the effects of smoking, including the cancer I just mentioned.

However, that does not give you a license to smoke. The tea detox can only help you so much.

Reduce Bad Breath

I've never met anyone who likes bad breath. Without a doubt, a stinky mouth is always an embarrassment when in public.

I have seen people restrain themselves from talking afraid of the bad air in their mouths. You don't need to be one of them. There is a better solution to this. And it's not breath mints or bubble gums.

I'm sure you have already guessed it – the tea detox.

Bad breath can be caused by many things. A clogged colon is among the causes.

With wastes building up in it, bacteria also increases. And this results in bad odor coming from the mouth.

You Get Healthy Hair

Hair means a lot more to women that men can understand. It's the reason most women spend a good proportion of their income on hair care products. But in some situations, the remedy might be to just get rid of toxins in the body.

Although this may not transform your hair like your favorite healthy care product, it will still have an effect in the long-term.

In addition to the detox, you should also drink more water. It also results in healthy hair.

Reduce the Risk of Heart Attack

This is among the leading killers in the world. But with a simple tea detox, you can reduce your chances of suffering from it.

Stop Premature Aging

Because of the toxins, we have unhealthy skins. And this is contributing to premature aging. With the teatox, you can keep yourself looking younger for quite some time.

Improved Sleep

With all sorts of toxins disrupting body processes, it's no wonder most of us fail to get a good night sleep. A less known benefit of detoxing is improved sleep.

Getting some shut eye is really important. It boosts immunity, makes you more productive, reduces stress, and a lot more benefits. And the best way to guarantee those benefits is to first clean your body.

Have Strong Bones

In a study, it was discovered that tea drinkers had stronger bones that those who do not drink tea. Since strength is something we all seek, this is an advantage you shouldn't ignore.

Boosts Brain Power

The cells housed in your skull are among the most important cells you have in your body. They control just about every process. And most importantly, they enable you to make sense of the world.

However, toxins can inhibit the growth of these cells. And sometimes, they may even destroy them. Destroyed cells mean decreased brain power.

But you can avoid that with a tea detox. Not only do the ingredients in tea protect brain cells from damage, but they also nourish them.

Tea is Hydrating

Forget the fact that there is caffeine in tea. It's small when you compare it with the amount of water in the tea.

Water is crucial for survival. Actually, your body is 60-70% water. If facing severe dehydration, cells can die.

The problem is that we don't usually drink enough water. But the teatox may give you a chance to drink enough of it.

Water helps you concentrate, reduce mood swings, increase energy, and a whole lot of other benefits.

Even better, is has been proven to increase metabolism.

Chapter 7: Why The Tea Cleanse Works

You may surely know a couple of detoxes that are even more popular than the tea cleanse. But then you would wonder what it is that makes the tea detox special.

If that sounds like you, this chapter will answer your questions. Here is why the tea cleanse works:

Tea Has a Lot of Antioxidants

Tea's biggest secret is the abundant antioxidants that it has. You may have heard that fruits and vegetables have more antioxidants. But here is a little news flash for you: green and black teas have 10 times the number of antioxidants in fruits and veggies.

Now you may be asking why these antioxidants are so special. Here are the reasons:

Speed metabolism – research has showed that the antioxidants in tea are responsible for speeding metabolism. This means that you would be able to burn a lot of fats. If you are trying to lose weight, you know how crucial this is. So even if you are just resting, you will still be using a lot of energy. In the end, you will use more calories and set yourself on the path to a healthy weight.

Eliminate free radicals – the simple process of getting oxygen into the body can destroy your life. The thing is that by taking in oxygen, you start the process of oxidation. This can destroy your cells as oxygen reacts with free radicals. You may end up with conditions like cancer and blood clots.

The antioxidants are there to destroy these free radicals.

The world's biggest tea drinkers, Japan and China, have fewer cases of most diseases and they also do not have certain types of cancers. All this is attributed to the presence of antioxidants.

Tea Is Low in Calories

Another thing that makes the tea cleanse a better option is that tea is low in calories. And as you may already know, having excess calories is what causes weight gain. So clearly, by following this diet, you should be able to lose some weight.

Encourages You to Eat Healthy Food

When you are on the tea cleanse, you are advised to eat healthy food. Not only does this give you enough nutrients, but it also provides you with a lot of fiber, something instrumental in cleaning the body.

Readily Available

Another reason to go for the tea detox is because tea is easy to find. Also, it's cheaper. This may not be the case with other detox diets.

Chapter 8: Why The Tea Cleanse Is Better Than Other Detoxes

There are a lot of detoxes out there you can take to clean your body. But by far, the teatox is among the best you can have.

Here are some of the reasons why that is so:

It Promotes Healthy Eating – As you saw in the book, by taking the tea cleanse, you will learn how to eat healthily. Unlike other detoxes, the teatox does not force you to give up foods you need to survive.

Instead, you get a list of foods you must eat along with the tea. Not only will this keep you from starving yourself, but you will also be getting all the nutrients you need on a daily basis. So if you thought that this is another detox that will leave you crawling on your stomach, you have been wrong.

No Side Effects – Giving up on foods you should be eating every day comes at a price. With most detoxes, you will experience headaches, fatigue, low concentration, and other signs.

But when you do the tea cleanse, since you still get all the food you need, you do not get any of those effects. Although you may be forbidden from eating your favorite foods, you will still not face the consequences of starvation.

It is Cheaper When Compared to Other Detoxes – Take the Juicing detox for example. You will first need to buy a juicer and then start buying fruits and vegetables. All this will cost you a lot of money. And even then, we all know that it is better to eat your fruits and vegetables than to drink them.

So when you look at the tea detox, you will realize that it is cheaper. You do not need to make huge investments as with other diets. The ingredients you need to get started are readily available.

Easy to Follow – Detoxes are a hell of a ride especially for the first time. But when we are talking about the tea cleanse, the story is different. All you need is tea and some healthy foods. What else could be so easy to understand or follow than that.

Chapter 9: Issues To Consider Before You Do The Tea Cleanse

The tea cleanse is as good as it sounds. But before you happily jump on it, you must ensure that you have taken some things into account. Failure to do so can make you become a victim of something with the potential of changing your life.

From the previous chapter, you already know why the tea detox is better than other detoxes. But here are some issues that may make you think twice before you adopt it:

Some Tea Detoxes Will Render Your Contraceptives Useless – If you decide to go for a tea manufactured by some company, make sure that you read everything before you use the tea. Although you will have some quick instructions on the box, they are not always enough. If the manufacturer has a website, visit it and read everything about the tea. If you still have questions, contact the manufacturer.

A certain woman reported using a detox tea without knowing that she risked becoming pregnant. Unfortunately, this info was not indicated on the packaging. It was hidden in the disclaimer section of the website.

Look at The Ingredients – If you are making the tea yourself and not buying it from a manufacturer, it means you will know everything you will throw in it.

But if you buy it already manufactured, you must determine what has gone into it.

Some manufacturers use herbs to boost the effectiveness of their teas. Unfortunately, you may be allergic to these herbs, which makes using the tea risky.

You Have Other Conditions – if you have some kind of a disease or are pregnant, it is advisable that you first talk to your doctor before taking a tea cleanse. As the old saying goes, it is better to be safe than sorry. Just because something has potential to improve your life doesn't mean you can just take it.

Detoxes Are Yet to Be Backed by Medical Research – One thing you must know is that detoxes are yet to be backed by medical science. Research is being conducted to establish the authenticity of using detoxes.

But by using logic, you would see how a tea cleanse is important. It encourages you to take lots of tea, which is high in antioxidants and eat other healthy foods. So who needs science to determine that this is something beneficial for him.

Chapter 10: Which Teas To Drink

We are all different, and so, have different tastes. The tea cleanse diet gives you a lot of options on the types of teas that you can drink. If you thought you would be bored with this diet, you have been wrong. Furthermore, the huge range of options means you will easily find something that's plentiful in your area.

Below are some of the teas that you can use to cleanse your body:

Milk Thistle Tea – The liver is one of the most important organs when it comes to getting rid of wastes. So it makes sense to keep it in top shape as any disturbances can be dangerous. And talking about taking care of the liver, there is nothing better than milk thistle tea.

This tea has silymarin, a compound that protects the liver. Furthermore, it helps in getting rid of toxins from this important organ.

But this tea is not only good for the liver as it's also beneficial to the digestive system. And as you may already know, the way you digest your food can have an impact on your energy and how your body gets rid of toxins.

Garlic – Don't mind being the least kissable person on earth? Then get your mouth dirty with some garlic. Despite ruining your mouth, garlic is one superfood that will get your health in check and clear some toxins from your body.

By taking it as a tea, you will still be able to enjoy all of its benefits. And this is also helpful if you can't stand eating it raw. You can add as many garlic cloves as you want in your tea.

Green Tea – This is the tea most of us have grown up drinking. And it is the tea you will also find in most restaurants. As if not enough, it tastes great and is available almost anywhere.

Green tea is packed with a lot of antioxidants than you will find in carrots, broccoli, or spinach. These antioxidants are the ones responsible for cleaning the toxins in your body. They also increase metabolism so that you can burn more calories and lose weight.

If you find that you need to enhance the taste of your tea even further, you can add some lemons. Just make sure that you avoid adding a lot of sugar.

Red Clover Tea – This has been used in China to cure different diseases for a long time. And if you can drink it as tea, you will be guaranteed that you will lose some toxins.

Red clover tea is also loaded with a lot of antioxidants. It also has vitamin C and B. Even better, you can find it almost anywhere.

Chamomile Tea – This is one of the most popular tea detox herbals that you can take. Not only is it good for cleaning your body, but it also helps you prevent diseases like colds.

Chamomile tea soothes the way for a liver detox. And as I already said, it is important that you are in the forefront of helping your body get rid of toxins by assisting the liver.

Ginger tea – You may not love its taste, but you will need to drink it for the benefits it brings to your body. Ginger is one herb that has been used for a long time to treat a number of diseases.

And when it comes to cleaning your body, it is also known as one of the best cleansing herbs that there is.

Ginger is known to inhibit the growth of cancer cells. In addition to that, it helps in improving circulation, thereby making sure that the body gets rid of the poisons.

Apart from that, ginger is also great for the digestive system.

Japanese Matcha Tea – If you want a tea that will clean your body and make you feel like a newborn, then get yourself a packet of Matcha Tea. Actually, a single cup of this tea is equal to 10 cups of green tea. So if the later is already great, imagine what the former will do to you; it is chock-full of antioxidants.

But Matcha Tea does not only clean your body. It also prevents heart disease as it lowers LDL. In addition to that, it increases fat burning, meaning you lose more fat even when you are just seated.

Chapter 11: How To Do The Tea Cleanse

Now that you have a good understanding of what the tea cleanse is all about, it's time to look at how you can take it. The best part with this detox is that it is easy to follow and understand. Not only that, but it also promotes the eating of healthy food.

Following the Tea Cleanse

Doing the tea detox is easy. You first need to acquire a tea you believe is suitable for you. We already talked about the various types of teas you can take in the previous chapter. If you need a reminder, just go back.

If you buy your tea from a manufacturer, you will get instructions on how you can take it. If there are no instructions, however, keep on reading.

Soon after Waking Up - it is recommended that you boil some water and drink it before you eat anything. This is important as it gets your body ready for the cleanse you are about a to do. To increase the taste of the water, you can add some slices of lemons.

Breakfast - After 20-30 minutes, you should take your tea. If you want, you can add some herbs to ensure that your body gets the vitamins and antioxidants needed. The perfect tea to take in the morning is Matcha Tea. Its abundant antioxidants make it a winner.

During the Day - For the duration of the day, you can take as many cups of tea as you wish. This is unlike other detoxes which promote fasting for a better cleanse. 3 – 6 cups is usually all you need. Tea is low in calories, so no need to worry about gaining weight.

It is not necessary to restrict yourself to one kind of tea.

At Night - When you are done conquering what the day had to offer, you must do the colon cleanse.

This is nothing more than what it sounds like; getting rid of toxins in your colon. For the best results, you must add senna leaf in your tea as it has a laxative effect. If you want, you can also add other herbs.

For How Long Should You Do a Tea Cleanse

Now you may be wondering for how long you will need to do the tea cleanse. The answer is simple.

If you are just getting started, do not be tempted to do it for longer, you will need to start small. So doing it for 7 days is a good start.

When you get used to it, you can start doing it for 14 or even 28 days.

It is recommended that you detox at least twice per year.

Foods To Eat

Since you will be cleaning your body, you do not want to be adding in more garbage right away. So if you love pancakes, hamburgers, and similar foods, you will not find the teatox very fun.

Here is what you will need to eat.

Fruits and Vegetables – These two are foods that are heavily promoted to those who are doing the tea cleanse. However, you will need to avoid tropical fruits as they are full of sugar.

Fruits and veggies are filled with vitamins and antioxidants, things you need when you are cleaning your body.

So make sure that you are getting the recommended 6 servings of veggies per day and some fruits.

However, you must be cautious with what you add to your veggies when preparing them. Adding ingredients that are not healthy is counterproductive. If you can, eat raw. If that is not an option, consider boiling for just a minute.

Fats – Contrary to popular belief, fats are important in your diet. However, it's not all fats that are good for you. Some can wreck your healthy. So ensure that you are getting them from healthy sources like fish, olive oil, avocados, nuts, coconut oil, and more.

Proteins – Proteins must also be present in your diet. But again, only from healthy food. You can eat eggs, chicken, fish, beans, etc.

Carbohydrates – These are a fuel to your life's processes. So ensure that they are present in your diet. But again, you need to focus on the healthy ones. To simplify things, eat whole carbs and avoid their processed cousins.

Fiber – One thing people tend to ignore in their diets is fiber. But this is what makes you feel full. At the same time, it also aids in the movement of food, thereby helping you eliminate toxins. Good sources of fiber are vegetables, fruits, beans, and nuts.

Chapter 12: Making A Meal Plan

Even after knowing what to eat when detoxing, it can still be nerve-wracking to get started. How much food should you get? How much tea is enough for you?

In this chapter, I will teach you how to make a meal plan. Hopefully, this will ensure a smooth detox as you will have everything in place. Furthermore, you will discover ways of adding variety to your detox plan.

The Process of Making a Meal Plan

The actual process of making a meal plan is easy. You just need to know how it's done. Here are the steps you need to follow:

1. Know the Foods to Eat
In the last chapter, I gave foods you can eat when doing a tea detox.

Those foods will form the foundation of your plan. But you may discover that some of them are not available in your area. If so, seek other healthy alternatives.

2. Group the Foods
The list of foods to include in your diet can add up fast. And you will soon realize how overwhelming this can be. As a result, you may start skipping foods from other food groups.

A simple solution to this is to group your foods. Think of which ones are proteins, carbohydrates, fats, vegetables, and fruits.

3. Create Your Meal Plan
Having known and grouped your foods, you can proceed to create a meal plan. And this is easy. You must ensure that you are taking a food from each group. You need at least one food from each group daily.

As you can see, the tea detox is not like many detox plans.

This gives you the freedom to plan your own meals. You won't be forced to swallow anything you don't like. You are free to go any road you want as long as it's healthy.

4. Go Shopping
Your next task is to go shopping. The meal plan will give you a better idea of the quantity of food you need, reducing the risk of running out of food in the middle of your detox.

Sample Meal Plan

Here is a sample meal plan to give you an idea of how it looks like.

Breakfast – remember that with the tea detox, you will be waking up to a cup of tea. Also, whenever you get hungry, it's advisable to go for another cup of tea.

As for snacks, tea should be your number one option. But if you are looking for a change, you can have a fruit.

With that in mind, you are left to think of only lunch and dinner. Here is my sample plan for that:

Monday
Lunch: chickpea salad

Dinner: broiled salmon and brown rice

Tuesday
Lunch: tomato mozzarella sandwich

Dinner: grilled chicken, vegetables, and potatoes

Wednesday
Lunch: whole grain sandwich and vegetables

Dinner: basil shrimp summer salad and eggs

Thursday
Lunch: leftovers from the basil shrimp summer salad and eggs

Dinner: pizza and salad

Friday
Lunch: salad with tomatoes, olives, and cheese

Dinner: Souvlaki lamb and brown rice

Saturday
Lunch: whole grain sandwich and vegetables

Dinner: chickpea salad

Sunday

Lunch: leftovers from the chickpea salad and eggs

Dinner: turkey and artichoke sandwich

Chapter 13: Guide To Making Tea

Healthy is associated with tasteless food. It's also associated with being hungry most of the time. But that's true when we are talking about weight loss diets or other detoxes. When it comes to the tea detox, the story changes.

Not only do you enjoy a variety of healthy foods that are also delicious, but you also get to enjoy great tasting tea.

The thing is tea can taste great or horrible—it all depends on how you make it. In this chapter, I'll show you how to do it.

So without further ado, let's get to it.

Getting Tea

To have the best tea detox, you first need to get the right tea. I gave a list of some teas you can drink in chapter 5.

Whatever you choose, make sure it's of the best quality. That's your first guarantee that you will make great tea.

Once that is done, the next task is to keep the tea safe. Otherwise, it will degrade with time.

Tea must be kept it in an airtight container. Also, you must avoid exposing it to direct sunlight.

Making Tea

If you have everything in place, you then need to know how to make tea the right way.

1. First, you need water. But not just any water will do. For the best results, go for filtered or bottled water.

2. Boil the water – you must boil the water only once. Going beyond that will force most of the oxygen out. And your tea will taste flat.

3. Preheat cup – if you have hot water somewhere, it helps to pour it in the cup to preheat it. This keeps your tea from getting cold just after you pour it into the cup.

4. Add tea into Cup – once the cup is heated, you can get rid of the preheating water and add the tea into the cup. How much tea to use will depend on the type of tea you are using. If using tea bags, the rule is that one bag should go into one cup.

5. Pour boiling water into cup – with your tea in the cup, you can add the boiling water into it.

6. Let it steep – for the best results, you should give the tea enough time to steep. This will result in great tasting tea.

Usually, most teas have specific steeping times clearly stated. If yours doesn't, you can't go wrong with the old rule of 3-5 minutes.

7. Enjoy the tea.

This may seem like a lot of work, that's because it is. But that's the price you need to pay to have the best tea. And needless to say, the whole process will make your tea detox experience unforgettable.

Chapter 14: How To Ensure Success When Doing The Tea Cleanse

Nothing is more disappointing than taking the tea cleanse and see no change. To prevent that kind of a situation, I will give you some tips for success. Although these may seem insignificant, they carry a lot of weight.

Start Slow – Your first tea cleanse should not be your last; you must keep doing it from time to time. A common mistake, however, is to do it for longer than is necessary for a beginner. Although you can start with a 28-day tea cleanse, you should know that it is not advisable. Baby steps were made for a reason. So start small; your first one can last for 7 days.

Although this may not seem like much, it's better to start something and finish it. Your body will need to get used to the new eating patterns gradually.

Take Your Calendar into Consideration – If there is an oncoming event that may get in the way of your detox, your best option is to postpone the detox. Like I said, it's better to start something and finish it than quit midway.

So before you get on the teatox, take a look at your calendar.

You can start the tea cleanse on a weekend. Being at home means you will be in control of what you eat. (Just make sure your friends will not be visiting you with bottles of beer in hand).

Get Enough Sleep – Sleep is not just a recipe for babies grow faster. Getting some shut eye ensures that you give your body time to get rid of wastes.

In addition, sleeping for the recommended amount of time will ensure that you wake up energetic. So during the day, you will not have urges to reach for other foods to stay on your feet.

Listen to Your Body – While you are on the tea detox, you must pay attention to any warning signs coming from your body. Anything abnormal must not be ignored. The body is really good at sensing when something has gone wrong. So do not ignore what it is telling you.

If you feel strange, a quick search online should give you an idea of what you are experiencing. If the net does not provide you with satisfactory results, you may need to talk to your doctor.

Drink Water – This is the one thing you can abuse and still get rewarded for your actions. So drink lots of it every time. Besides, your body is made up of water so taking it in large quantities should not be a problem. You should drink at least 8 glasses per day.

Water plays a big role in cleaning your body.

Eat Fibrous Foods - another easy way to guarantee success when doing a tea detox is to eat fibrous foods. It's sad to see how devoid of fiber our diets are–we are so much into junk food. Making it worse, these junk foods increase the number of toxins in our bodies.

Fiber helps move things down the gut, thereby removing some of the wastes in your intestines.

Also, it makes you feel fuller for longer, making you eat less. If you are trying to lose weight, that's a plus.

Examples of fibrous foods include vegetables, fruits, and whole grains. You must incorporate these foods in your breakfasts, lunches, and dinners.

Do Light Exercises - detoxing doesn't mean you should abandon your workout routine. Exercising also helps get rid of wastes. So it makes sense to use it alongside the tea detox.

By exercising, you increase blood circulation. At the same time, you also amplify sweating and water intake. All these things are known to flush out toxins from the body.

The only problem is that you may be low on energy while detoxing. So a 5K run is not such a good idea. You will need to go for light exercises. Although these may not be as effective as intense ones, any workout is better than no workout.

Examples of light exercises include jogging, walking, cleaning the house, gardening, playing with kids, and cooking. Additionally, when at the office, you can try working while standing.

As for the duration of your exercises, that will depend on how busy you are and how much energy you have. But for you must aim for at least 30 minutes per day. If you can go for longer, that's even better. Just listen to your body for signs of exhaustion.

Plan - when on an important journey, you need to plan for how you will get to your destination. This includes working out the route, things to take, etc. Without a plan, you may end up being stranded in the middle of nowhere.

Cleaning your body is a big task. And it needs careful planning to ensure success.

Thankfully, planning for a tea detox is easy. You first need to have a goal, in this case, cleaning your body. With that, you need to think if you can achieve this. If yes, you should then make a strategy for achieving your goal. And lastly, you must get all the resources you need.

This book has all the tools for you to learn how to make a successful plan.

Meditate - it's not mandatory to meditate when doing the tea cleanse. But meditation may multiply the benefits of the detox.

Meditation calms your mind. And this reduces stress. As you may know, stress forces people to indulge in unhealthy habits. These may include smoking, alcohol drinking, and binge eating.

If you do not currently meditate, know that it's really simple. You just need to learn it from someone good at it. But for a start, there are a lot of guides teaching how to meditate on the internet. You can try using those.

Get Support - we are social animals. And we succeed in most things because of the support from family and friends.

So now that you are detoxing feel free to tell people around you about your cleanse.

If they do not understand what it's all about, tell them all about it. They may be interested in joining you. If not, then they will, at least, try to see that you are successful. For example, they will not force you to drink beer or smoke cigarettes.

Conclusion

The tea cleanse diet is a simple way to remove toxins from your body and improve your immune system. If you are feeling low and burdened, then try this diet because it will make you feel lighter and healthier. It will jump start your metabolism, turn on the hormones to trigger the fat-burning process. It will calm your body and mind while promoting your energy levels. If you are worried for your stubborn fat and unable to reduce your weight, then kick start your metabolism with the two weeks tea cleanse diet.

During this diet, you will strictly avoid sugar, fatty food, alcohol and other harmful food items. It is important to promote healthy weight loss and flush out harmful toxins from your body. It will surely improve metabolism and immune system of your body. If you are worried for your body fat, then it will be good to start this cleansing diet to have a flat belly. Green tea should be an important part of your diet because it will prove really helpful to reduce belly fat. You have to use some herbs and mix your green drinks with natural fruits. It will enable you to make delicious green smoothies and promote good health.

If you are suffering from high blood pressure, then this diet will help you to reduce blood pressure. You should avoid wheat, alcohol, caffeinated drinks and soft drinks to promote good health. You can do it for almost 14 days and then wait for three months to repeat it. With some exercise and diet control, you can retail this weight for a longer period of time. After starting this diet, you will start feeling lighter and healthier, even in the first week.

Thank you again for downloading this book!

www.ingramcontent.com/pod-product-compliance
Lightning Source LLC
Chambersburg PA
CBHW062136020426
42335CB00013B/1234